Gene Regulation

Edited by Payam Behzadi

Published in London, United Kingdom

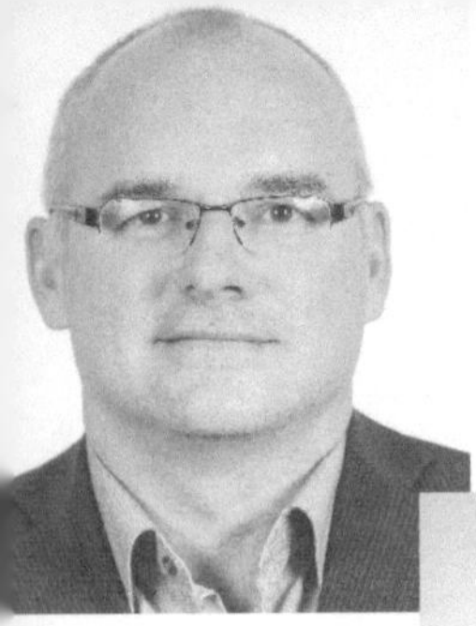
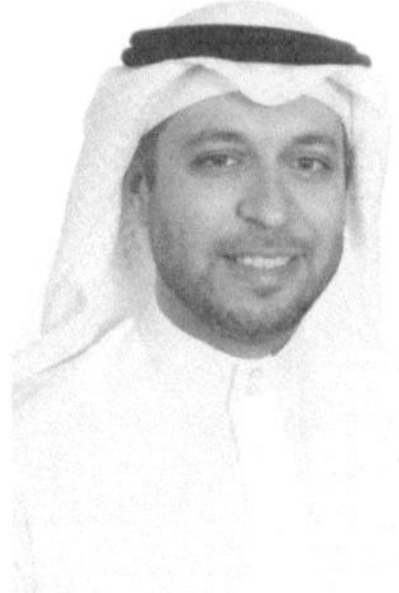
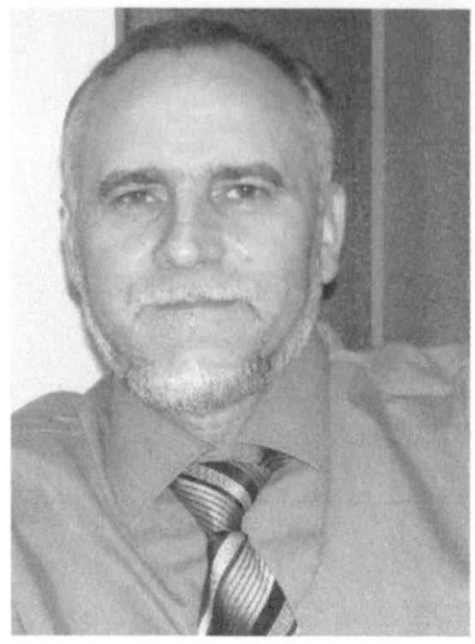
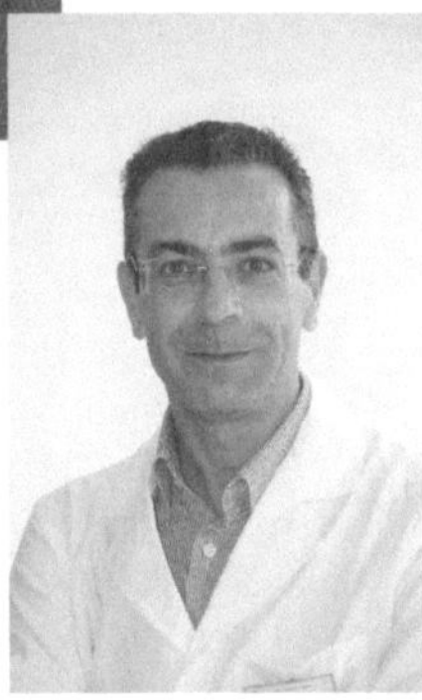
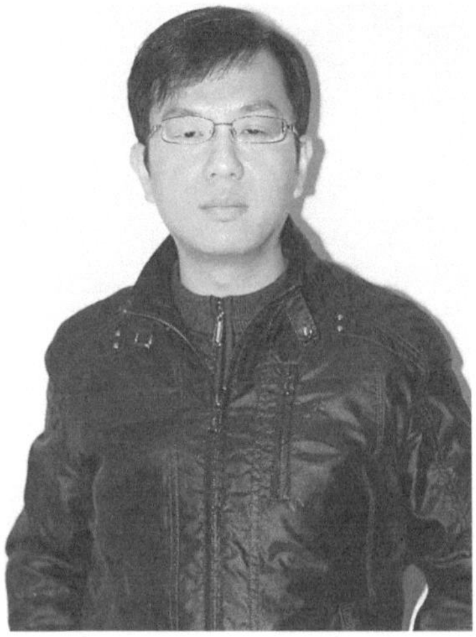
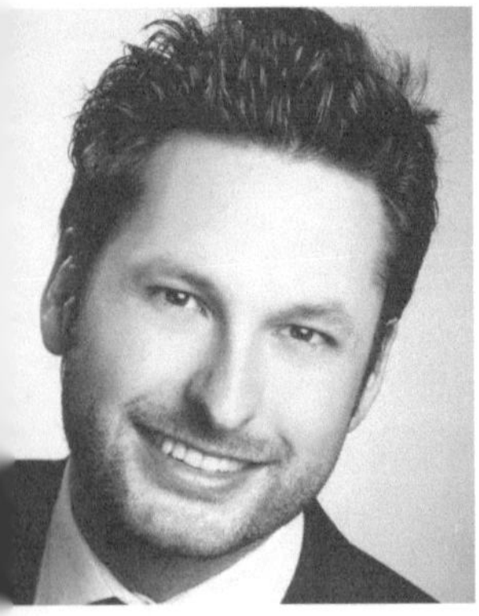
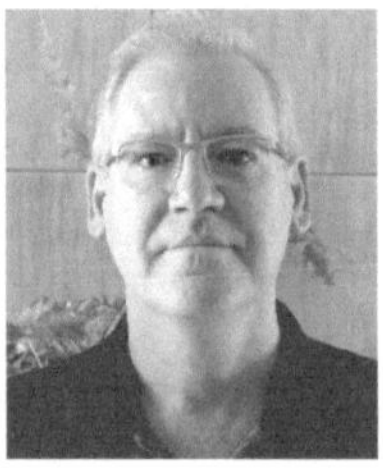

IntechOpen

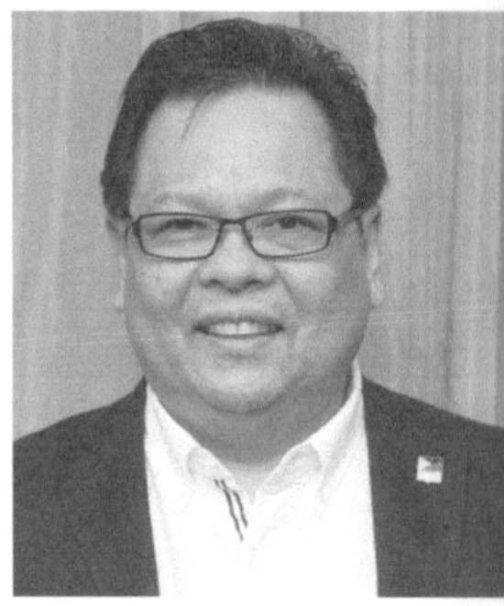
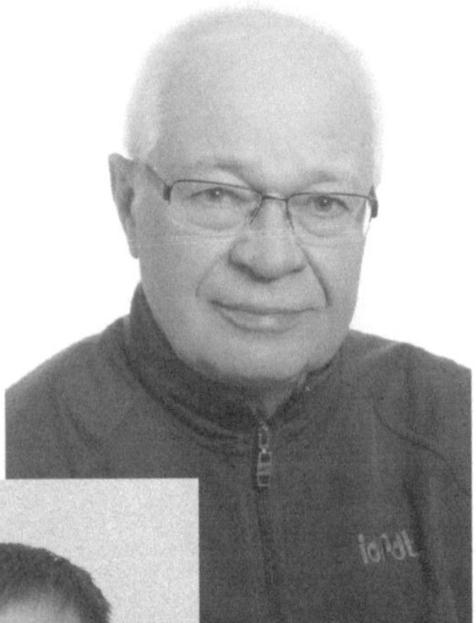
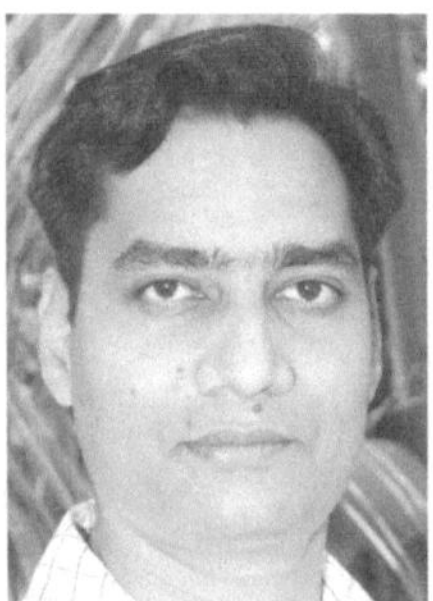
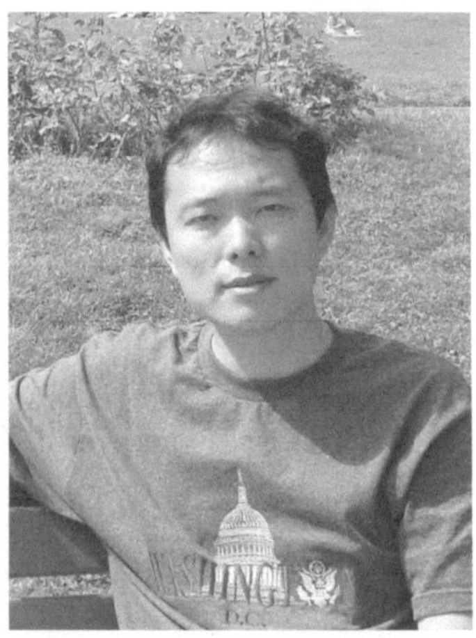
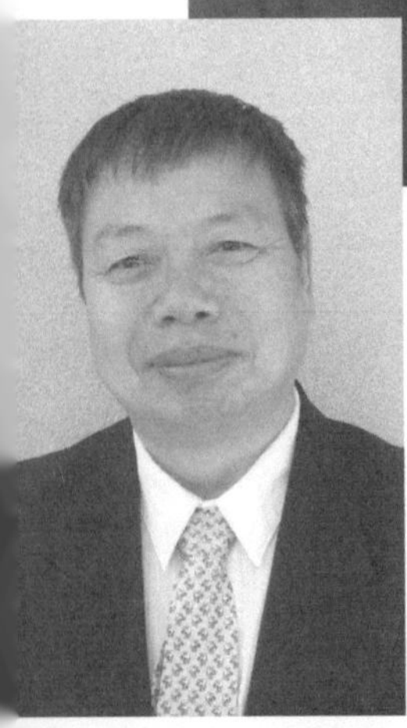
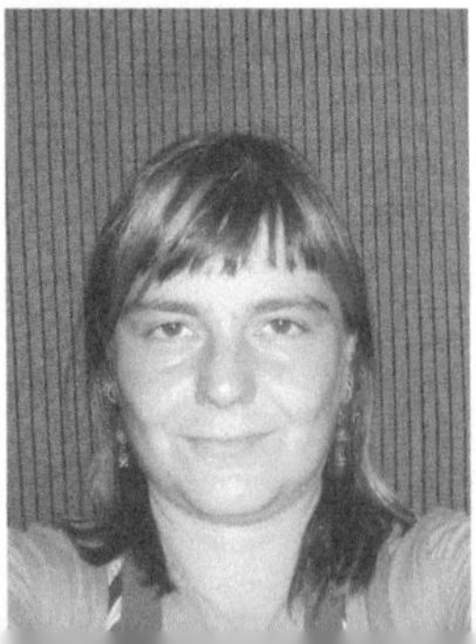

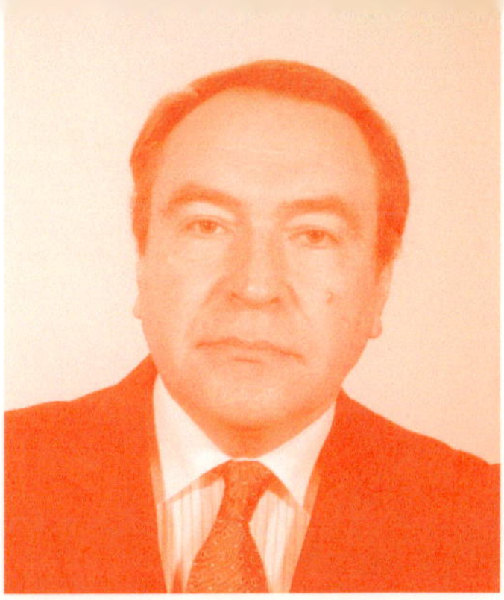
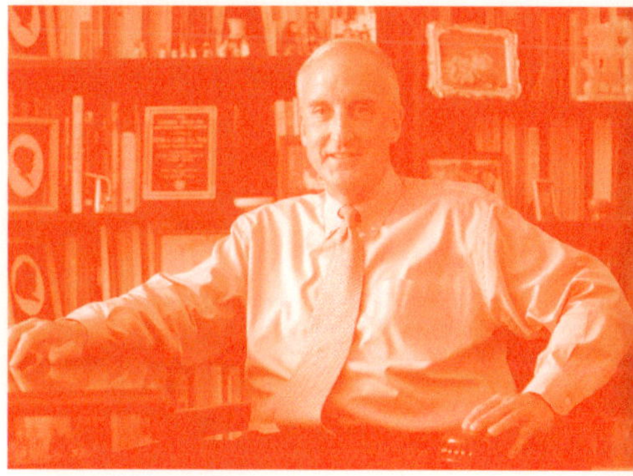
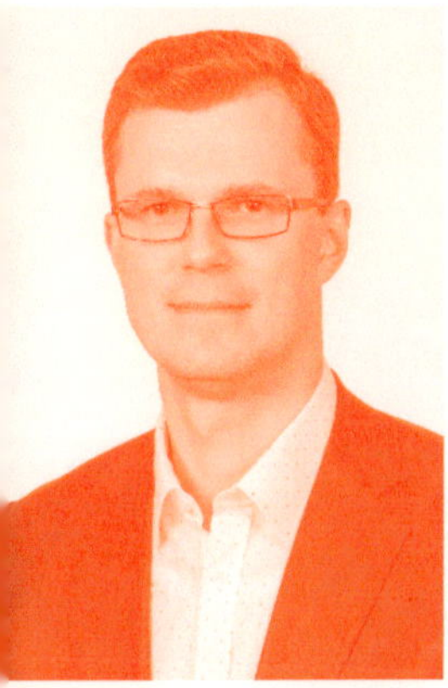
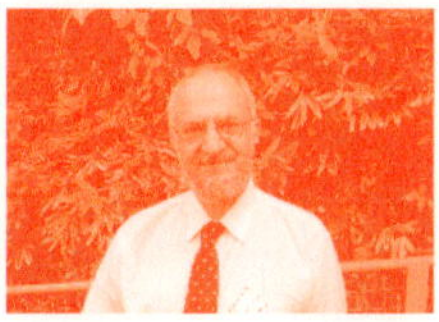
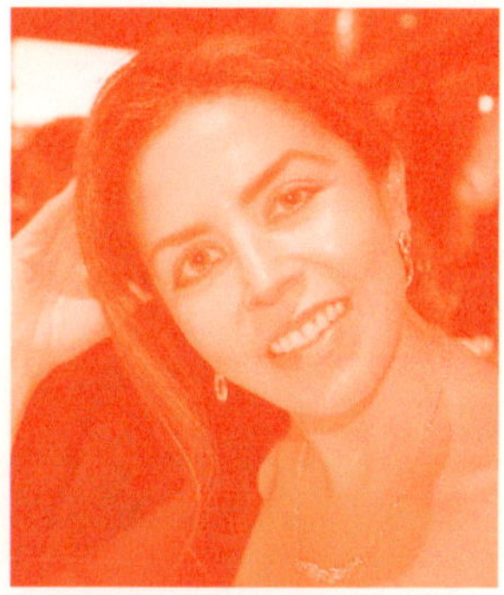

Supporting open minds since 2005

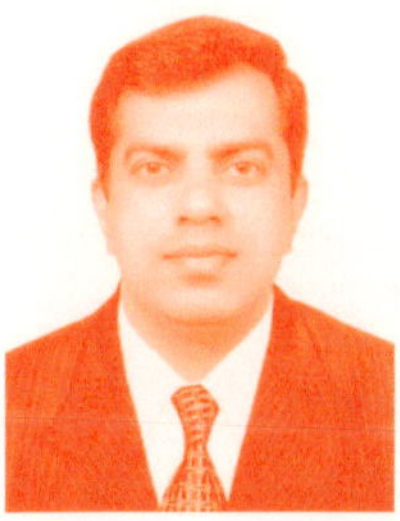
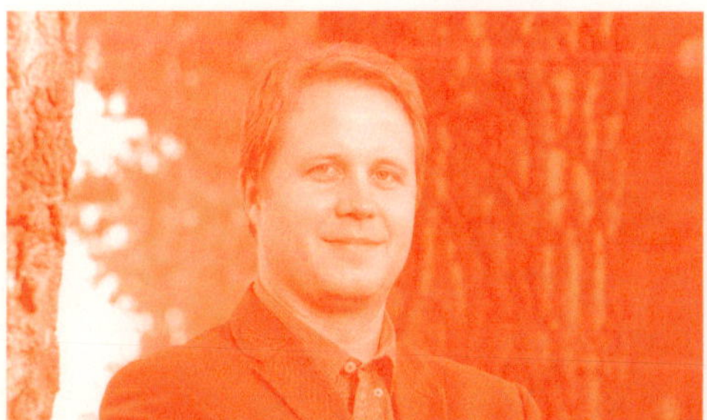
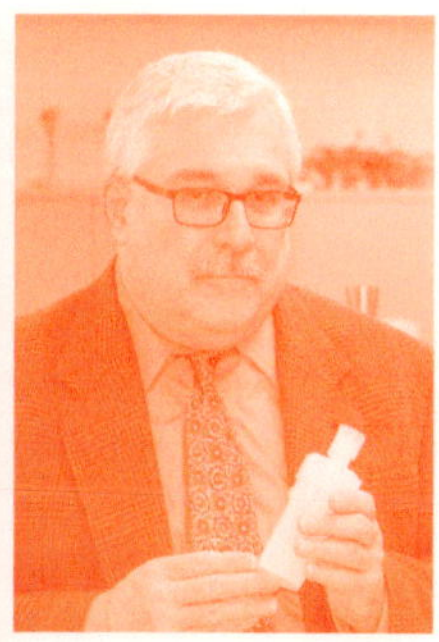
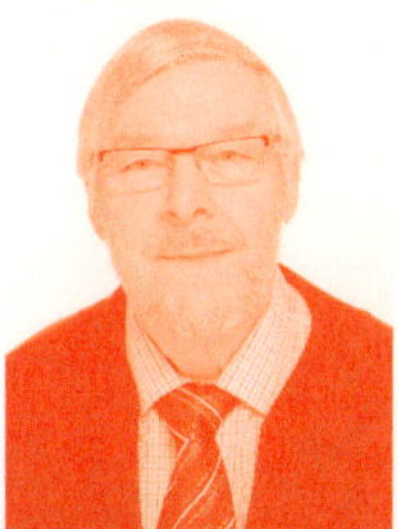
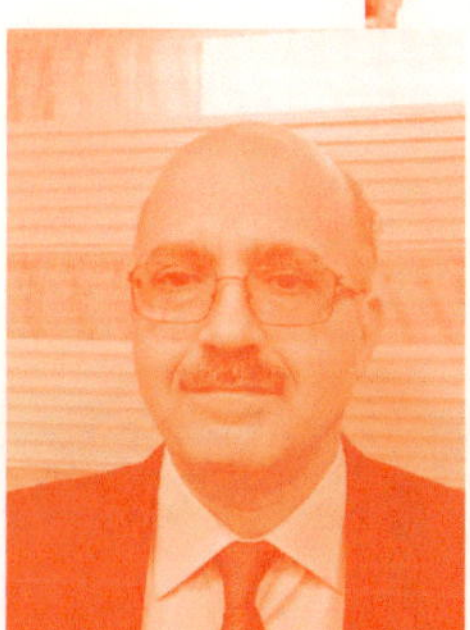
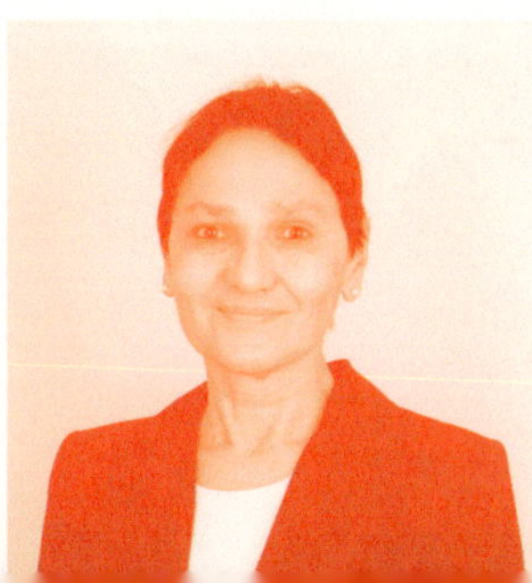
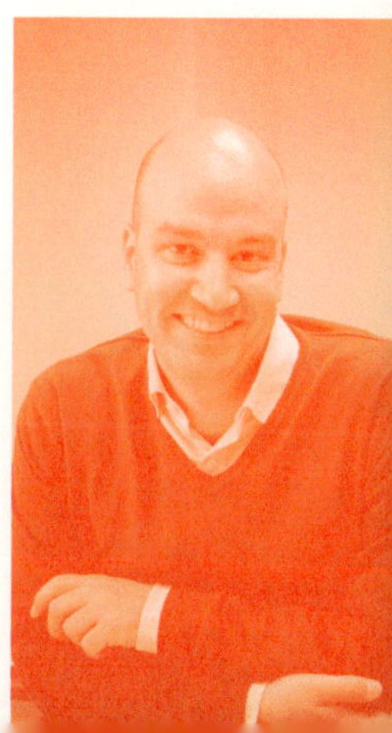

Gene Regulation
http://dx.doi.org/10.5772/intechopen.78432
Edited by Payam Behzadi

Contributors
Kiyoshi Ohtani, Hideyuki Komori, Ritsuko Iwanaga, Andrew Bradford, Keigo Araki, Felipe Garcia-Vallejo, Alejandra Rodriguez, Mailyn Bedoya, Julio Cesar Montoya, Thomas Meyer, Julia Staab, Roswitha Nast, Payam Behzadi, Lernik Issakhanian

First published in London, United Kingdom, 2019 by IntechOpen
IntechOpen is the global imprint of INTECHOPEN LIMITED, registered in England and Wales, registration number: 11086078, The Shard, 25th floor, 32 London Bridge Street
London, SE19SG – United Kingdom
Printed in Croatia

British Library Cataloguing-in-Publication Data
A catalogue record for this book is available from the British Library

Additional hard copies can be obtained from orders@intechopen.com

Gene Regulation
Edited by Payam Behzadi
p. cm.
Print ISBN 978-1-78985-683-5
Online ISBN 978-1-78985-684-2

Meet the editor

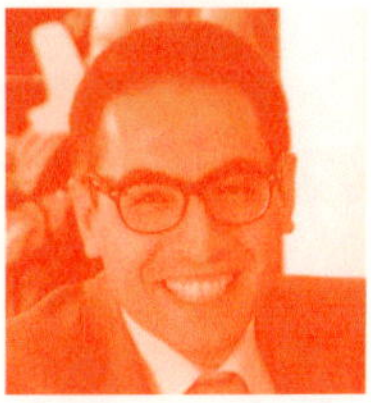

Dr. Payam Behzadi was born in 1973, Tehran, Iran. He began his collaboration with the Department of Microbiology, College of Basic Sciences, Shahr-e-Qods Branch, Islamic Azad University as a faculty member (with MSc degree in microbiology) in 2004. He received his PhD degree in molecular biology in 2016 (BSc and MSc in microbiology; PhD in molecular biology) and now continues his scientific activities in the position of Assistant Professor at the same university. He assists several students from different academic levels including BSc, MSc, and PhD. Dr. Payam Behzadi has authored and edited >15 chapters and academic books and >55 original and review articles. His scientific research interests are: urinary tract infections, bioinformatics, genetics, gene profiling, and molecular biology. Dr. Payam Behzadi trains as an ice skater in his free time.

Contents

Preface

Gene regulation is one of the most interesting and incredible discussion topics in life sciences. Indeed, the process of gene regulation is linked to many biomolecules, different spatial configuration of genes, enzymes, and environmental factors.

Genes are worthy pearls within the organisms' genomic treasure, which can be brightened in due course according to the needs of cells.

In recent years, by the progression of disciplines such as bioinformatics, computational biology, computational chemistry etc., our understanding of gene characteristics and gene regulation has been extended and is closer to natural processes. The main reason for this progression is the availability of the created 3-dimensional illustrations and animations thanks to advanced computational technologies, online and offline databases, tools, and software.

When we go back several decades, only DNA molecules were the cornerstone of gene regulation. Indeed, the network of DNA molecules was regarded as the center of the gene regulation process. Today, this point of view has changed. In recent years, the process of gene regulation is known as a twin structured composition in which both RNA and DNA molecules have a pivotal role. In other words, the feature of gene regulation is simultaneously processed by the complex system of RNA and DNA networks.

Although in parallel with DNAs, RNAs have a pivotal role in prokaryotic gene regulation and this feature is much bolder in Eukaryotes than in bacteria. Due to this fact, the size of eukaryotic genomes is much larger than prokaryotes and there are numerous RNAs that act as coding and noncoding RNAs (ncRNAs).

For example, the small nuclear RNAs (snRNAs) in Eukaryotes, which are situated in the nucleus, have a key role in the process of splicing, which may lead to formation of spliceosomes. This example is known as a normal process in eukaryotes and it does not occur in prokaryotic bacteria. Moreover, the process of splicing, which directly affects gene expression, separates the stages of transcription and translation in eukaryotes while the lack of splicing process in bacteria leads to simultaneous transcription and translation phases.

There are many examples that show the abundance of treasures relating to coding and ncRNAs in eukaryotes, which have a key role in the process of gene regulation.

In this regard, the presence of small RNAs of interference RNAs (RNAi) is an important occurrence in the post-transcriptional process that may lead to suppression or silencing gene expression. Interestingly, there are huge numbers of RNAi molecules with different mechanisms in different organisms.

Despite limited information regarding RNAi molecules, it is known that they are vital molecules that affect the process of gene regulation by controlling and/or determining the expression of the genes. The RNAi molecules act as gene silencers by translation inhibition and/or degradation of RNAs (mostly mRNAs).

All in all, the ncRNAs, rather than coding RNAs, contribute in the process of gene suppression, gene expression, and *in toto*, gene regulation. That's why the RNA network, in parallel with the DNA network, contributes to gene regulation.

In this book, different authors from different countries have presented their invaluable knowledge. Each chapter has its individual scientific worth and importance. Therefore, I suggest to scientists who work in the fields of genes, molecular biology and genetics not to miss this practical information. This book contains worthy information for its readers!

With Best Wishes
Payam BEHZADI
Assistant Professor,
Department of Microbiology,
College of Basic Sciences,
Shahr-e-Qods Branch,
Islamic Azad University,
Tehran, Iran

Chapter 1

Introductory Chapter: Gene Regulation, an RNA Network-Dependent Architecture

Payam Behzadi and Lernik Issakhanian

1. A historical background of genetics

Genetics is known as an old and ancient science that its origination goes back to at least 7000 years ago. Iranians are one of the earliest pioneers in genetics from ancient world. The brilliant Iranian (Persian) literature epic of *Shahnameh* edited by the Iranian shining star literate "Abolqasem Ferdowsi Toosi" is an invaluable evidence to prove this claim. By the time and progression in biology, the super-amazing molecule of DNA was discovered. Today, we know that the unique molecule of DNA involves the genetic and vital data within its bases as constitutional structures of nucleotides. Both eukaryotic and prokaryotic chromosomes are made up of DNA molecules. In addition to DNAs, the role and importance of RNAs are not lesser than DNAs [1].

In 1953, the interesting structure of DNA molecule with anti-parallel double-helix architecture was recognized by Watson and Crick. In 1958, the hypothesis of central dogma of molecular biology was published by Crick in which he described the translation of genetic language located on DNA into amino acid sequences of protein by the transient molecule of RNA (mainly messenger RNA (mRNA)). The primitive biological characteristics of mRNA were recognized in 1961, while these properties regarding ribosomal RNA (rRNA) and transfer RNA (tRNA) molecules were determined in the 1950s [2].

2. Central dogma

In accordance with central dogma of molecular biology, the genetic information hidden in the format of gene can be expressed throughout two vital processes of transcription (production of coding molecules of mRNA) and translation (in which nucleotides are replaced by amino acids). The central dogma's content involves both eukaryotes and prokaryotes. In this regard, the RNA polymerase (RNAP) contributes in the process of transcription to produce mRNA molecules from DNAs. In the process of translation, ribosomes are also contributed. As it is known, the eukaryotic processes of transcription and translation are separated; this separation is because of the presence of intron sequences among exons. Indeed, introns were discovered in 1977 in eukaryotes which resulted in the recognition of their localization among exon sequences. In other words, the arrangement of introns was revealed as noncoding mosaics of introns among the coding mosaics of exons. Normally introns, dependent on the eukaryotic cell's need, should be eliminated via the splicing process. The splicing process, which leads to the occurrence of the spliceosome, separates the direct connection between transcription and translation stages, while the bacterial system misses splicing process. Therefore, the processes of transcription and translation couple together in bacteria. Furthermore, the coupling system of transcription-translation is achieved via the functional enzyme complex of RNAP and ribosome which is known as expressosome in bacteria [2–4].

Amazingly, the ribozyme domains (e.g. small self-cleaving RNAs) are present in noncoding sequences of introns and untranslated regions (UTRs) (mostly in 3′UTRs) [2, 5].

By the progression of knowledge and technology from the 1970s in the twentieth century, the importance of the role of RNA molecules increased more and more. Pre-mRNA molecules in eukaryotes which are known as heterogeneous nuclear RNA (hnRNA) have incredible role in gene regulation and expression. Different manners for the beginning of transcription, different patterns of splicing process, different lengths of poly-adenine tails and different patterns in RNA editing processes have direct effects on gene regulation and expression. Incredibly, the RNA molecules act as *trans*-acting factors that affect the processes of gene regulation and gene expression [6, 7].

These characteristics relating to RNAs support the RNA World Hypothesis (RWH). According to RWH which was proposed by Alex Rich, RNAs are bifunctional biopolymers which can appear in two different levels of bioactivities including enzymatic activities (ribozymes) and as informational genetic language. However, the Urzymes hypothesis challenges RWH. Urzymes are the earliest generation of enzymes originated from protein superfamilies with a conserved nucleus [6, 8–10].

The progression of the Internet, computers and online/offline software and tools, bioinformatics and computational biology and chemistry gives us a new horizon in association with gene, gene regulation, gene expression and gene structure. By the help of advanced knowledge and technology, now it is known that DNA molecules play their roles as CDs which are burned and contain cells' software tools as genetic information which encode into RNAs and proteins [1, 11].

3. RNA molecules, RNA network and gene regulation

In recent years throughout very strong evidences, it has revealed that the RNA molecules are not only temporal and transient transcripts which are obtained from the genes, but also they act as pivotal modulators that mediate pre-transcriptional and posttranscriptional steps and have direct effect on gene regulation and gene expression processes. Also, RNA molecules play a key role in producing and triggering vital signals within the wide web of genomic structure. Now, it is known that there are two main groups of coding RNA and noncoding RNA (ncRNA) molecules in which each of them has its own functions, structures and characteristics. The coding RNA molecules are those which can be translated into proteins, while the ncRNAs cannot be translated in proteins. According to previous studies, a large group of RNAs has no ability to be translated. And in mammals as an important group of eukaryotes, only less than 2% of the transcribed RNA molecules can be translated into protein molecules. So, the population of ncRNAs overpasses the population of coding RNAs [1, 2, 6, 12, 13].

RNAs are important allosteric molecules that regulate the processes of gene regulation and gene expression. The allosteric property of RNAs enables them to switch different pathways by regulation of genes to be expressed or silenced. A great cooperation among rRNAs, tRNAs, mRNAs and small nuclear RNAs (snRNAs) in the processes of eukaryotic transcription and translation explains the depth of the RNA roles within a cell. In addition, eukaryotes encompass small nucleolar RNAs (snoRNAs), too. snoRNAs with 60–300 nucleotide lengths are known as intermediate size of ncRNAs. They have different roles including targeting a diversity of RNA molecules such as mRNA. This property depicts the regulatory role of snoRNAs. In this regard, there is another group of snRNAs known as small Cajal body-specific RNAs (scaRNAs) located in Cajal bodies or coiled bodies (CBs). CBs are compact organelles which are recognized within the eukaryotic nuclei. The CBs are consisted of a mass of proteins including snRNPs and snoRNPs. scaRNAs and snoRNAs are significant molecules which contribute in processing and modification of other RNA molecules like mRNA, rRNA, tRNA and snRNA. Interestingly, rRNAs are remarkable molecules which constitute ribosomal peptidyl transferase site. This illustrates the important role of RNAs as ribozymes which contribute in activation of peptidyl transferring and constitution of peptide bonds within polypeptides. Today it is known that short ncRNAs (such as microRNAs (miRNAs), Piwi-interacting RNAs (piRNAs), transcription initiation RNAs (tiRNAs)), promoter-associated RNAs (PARs) (including promoter-associated small RNAs (PASRs), transcriptional start site-associated RNAs (TSSa-RNAs) and promoter upstream transcripts (PROMPTS)) and long noncoding RNAs (lncRNAs) (comprising large intergenic noncoding RNAs (lincRNAs), transcribed ultraconserved regions (T-UCRs), telomeric repeat-containing RNAs (TERRAs), etc.) have unique role in gene regulation and gene expression [1, 2, 6, 14–19].

In prokaryotes such as bacteria, a diversity of small RNAs (sRNAs) act as regulatory molecules. These molecules are contributed in gene regulation and gene expression. Moreover, the *cis*-acting sequences of regulatory RNAs which are known as riboswitches have an effective role on gene regulation. In addition, some special DNA sequences have been recognized in bacteria and archaea which are known as clustered regulatory interspaced short palindromic repeats (CRISPRs). CRISPERs are able to be transcribed. The processed CRISPR transcripts act as guide RNAs (gRNAs) which destruct the viral nucleic acids including RNA or DNA molecules [2].

4. The importance and the role of NCRNA molecules

The ncRNAs are divided into two groups of lncRNAs (with >200 nucleotide lengths) and small ncRNAs (sncRNAs) (with 20–35 nucleotide lengths). Among different types of sncRNAs, the miRNAs are well-studied RNAs. They belong to RNA interference (RNAi) members with the length of 19–24 nucleotides. Amazingly, >60% of the coding genes are regulated by miRNAs. In other words, these molecules contribute in posttranscriptional process by silencing the related genes by prevention of translation. Drosha and Dicer are key enzymes to manufacture a mature miRNA molecule. The linkage of a single-stranded miRNA with the members of Argonautes produces RNA-induced silencing complex (RISC). The RISC binds to its complementary sequence on the 3′UTR section of targeted mRNA. In addition to miRNA pathway, piRNA and siRNA pathways are members of RNAi pathways. piRNAs (with about 30 nucleotide lengths) and siRNAs resembling miRNAs bind to Argonautes to produce RISCs which contribute in gene silencing process. However, miRNAs have genomic origination, while the siRNAs may have exo- or endogenous origination. The piRNAs are free dicer pathways which bind to PIWI proteins. The PIWI proteins are known as the subset of Argonautes. The complex of PIWI proteins and piRNAs contributes in transposon repression via degradation of transcripts belonging to transposable elements (epigenetic regulation). Furthermore, the piRNAs mediate the DNA methylation too. The tiRNAs as members of sncRNAs with about 17 nucleotide lengths may act as transcriptional regulators [1, 13, 18, 20, 21].

snoRNAs contribute in rRNA modification within the nucleolus. These modifications involve pseudouridylation and 2'-O-methylation of rRNAs to promote the integrity and rRNA folding. According to characterizations of secondary structure and common motifs, the snoRNAs are divided into two main families of box C/D and box H/ACA. Interestingly, the majority of snoRNA molecules are mostly expressed from housekeeping gene introns. The presence of abundance of snRNAs and scaRNAs support the rate of snRNA modification [2, 16, 18].

PASRs (with 22–200 nucleotide lengths), PROMPTs (with lesser than 200 nucleotides in length) and TSSa-RNAs (with 20–90 nucleotide lengths) are categorized within the intermediate ncRNAs in size and have not been studied well [18].

The lncRNAs are consisted of heterogeneous ncRNAs with the length of >200 nucleotides. They are known as the dominant mammalian ncRNAs of transcriptome. lncRNAs are recognized as effective eukaryotic ncRNAs with a wide range of functions. lncRNAs are involved in gene expression and gene regulation by regulating the posttranscriptional processes, epigenetic modifications, etc. [2, 18, 22].

In conclusion, we can claim that RNA molecules have a key role in molecular biology. In recent years, the sciences of bioinformatics, computational biology and computational chemistry have offered us a new promise regarding the importance of RNAs in association with gene regulation.

Acknowledgements

We have special thanks to Lada BOZIC, the author service manager of InTechOpen Company for her excellent collaboration, management and arrangement for preparing this valuable book.

Conflict of interest

The authors declare no conflicts of interest.

Author details

Payam Behzadi[1]* and Lernik Issakhanian[2]

1 Department of Microbiology, College of Basic Sciences, Shahr-e-Qods Branch, Islamic Azad University, Tehran, Iran

2 Independent Researcher, PCR Specialist, Yerevan, Armenia

*Address all correspondence to: behzadipayam@yahoo.com

References

[1] Behzadi P, Behzadi E, Ranjbar R. Basic Modern Molecular Biology. 1st ed. Tehran: Persian Science & Research Publisher; 2014

[2] Morris KV, Mattick JS. The rise of regulatory RNA. Nature Reviews. Genetics. 2014;**15**(6):423

[3] Klaholz BP. The ribosome holds the RNA polymerase on track in bacteria. Trends in Biochemical Sciences. 2017;**42**(9):686-689

[4] Kohler R, Mooney R, Mills D, Landick R, Cramer P. Architecture of a transcribing-translating expressome. Science. 2017;**356**(6334):194-197

[5] De La Peña M, García-Robles I. Intronic hammerhead ribozymes are ultraconserved in the human genome. EMBO Reports. 2010;**11**(9):711-716

[6] Licatalosi DD, Darnell RB. Resolving RNA complexity to decipher regulatory rules governing biological networks. Nature Reviews. Genetics. 2010;**11**(1):75

[7] Bass BL. RNA editing by adenosine deaminases that act on RNA. Annual Review of Biochemistry. 2002;**71**(1):817-846

[8] Neveu M, Kim H-J, Benner SA. The "strong" RNA world hypothesis: Fifty years old. Astrobiology. 2013;**13**(4):391-403

[9] Li L, Francklyn C, Carter CW. Aminoacylating urzymes challenge the RNA world hypothesis. Journal of Biological Chemistry. 2013;**288**(37):26856-26863

[10] Carter CW. Urzymology: Experimental access to a key transition in the appearance of enzymes. Journal of Biological Chemistry. 2014;**289**(44):30213-30220

[11] Omoto CK, Lurquin P, Lurquin PF. Genes and DNA: A Beginner's Guide to Genetics and its Applications. New York, United States: Columbia University Press; 2004

[12] Fatica A, Bozzoni I. Long non-coding RNAs: New players in cell differentiation and development. Nature Reviews. Genetics. 2014;**15**(1):7

[13] Bunch H. Gene regulation of mammalian long non-coding RNA. Molecular Genetics and Genomics. 2018;**293**(1):1-15

[14] Bandyra K, Luisi B. Central dogma alchemy. RNA. 2015;**21**(4):558-559

[15] Ronchetti D, Todoerti K, Tuana G, Agnelli L, Mosca L, Lionetti M, et al. The expression pattern of small nucleolar and small Cajal body-specific RNAs characterizes distinct molecular subtypes of multiple myeloma. Blood Cancer Journal. 2012;**2**(11):e96

[16] Meier UT. RNA modification in Cajal bodies. RNA Biology. 2017;**14**(6):693-700

[17] Xie J, Zhang M, Zhou T, Hua X, Tang L, Wu W. Sno/scaRNAbase: A curated database for small nucleolar RNAs and cajal body-specific RNAs. Nucleic Acids Research. 2006;**35**(suppl_1):D183-D1D7

[18] Esteller M. Non-coding RNAs in human disease. Nature Reviews. Genetics. 2011;**12**(12):861

[19] Darzacq X, Jády BE, Verheggen C, Kiss AM, Bertrand E, Kiss T. Cajal body-specific small nuclear RNAs: A novel class of 2′-O-methylation and pseudouridylation guide RNAs. The EMBO Journal. 2002;**21**(11):2746-2756

[20] Wilson RC, Doudna JA. Molecular mechanisms of RNA interference.

Annual Review of Biophysics. 2013;**42**:217-239

[21] Ku H-Y, Lin H. PIWI proteins and their interactors in piRNA biogenesis, germline development and gene expression. National Science Review. 2014;**1**(2):205-218

[22] Bánfai B, Jia H, Khatun J, Wood E, Risk B, Gundling WE, et al. Long noncoding RNAs are rarely translated in two human cell lines. Genome Research. 2012;**22**(9):1646-1657

Chapter 2

Temporal and Spatial Differential Expression of Glutamate Receptor Genes in the Brain of Down Syndrome

Alejandra Rocio Rodríguez Ortiz, Mailyn Alejandra Bedoya Saldarriaga, Julio César Montoya Villegas and Felipe García-Vallejo

Abstract

Studying the dysregulation of expression of glutamate receptors is crucial to better understand the mechanisms associated with cognitive disabilities in Down syndrome (DS) patients. By using data of microarray experiments previously deposited in GEO Dataset, we studied the expression of 26 glutamate receptor genes in DS brain samples since prenatal to adult age in several brain structures. Overall, our results showed a complexity in the expression of the genes which were dependent mainly on the brain structure analyzed; especially, the hippocampus showed a different expression pattern. While in the general brain analysis the overexpressed genes were GRIN3A and GRIN2C, higher expression levels of GRM1, GRID2, and GRIK1 gene receptors were recorded in hippocampus. Our results suggest that the glutamatergic system in association with other neurotransmitter systems in the human brain would associate with glutamatergic receptor alterations to bring upon synaptic changes and cognitive deficits in DS models.

Keywords: glutamatergic system, gene expression, Down syndrome, brain, bioinformatics

1. Introduction

Down syndrome (DS) or trisomy 21 is the leading cause of genetically defined intellectual disability, developmental brain abnormalities, and congenital birth defects. The phenotypical features of this syndrome affect almost all body systems, including neurodevelopment and cognitive aspects [1, 2]. Brains of individuals with DS show decreased volume and reduced neuronal density in diverse areas including the cortex, hippocampus, and cerebellum [3–7], leading to delayed cognitive progress in infancy and childhood and mild-to-moderate intellectual disability [8–11]. Also, during adulthood, there is a loss of cognitive abilities and the development of Alzheimer's disease (AD) by the fourth decade of life [12, 13]. Glutamate is the principal and main excitatory neurotransmitter in the body [14–16]. Glutamate receptors are classified into metabotropic—G-coupled protein receptors—and ionotropic—ligand-gated ion channels [17–26]. Many studies have agreed that a major function of glutamate receptors is the modulation of synaptic plasticity, which is the ability of neurons to change its connections in response to a stimuli; this mechanism is thought to be vital for memory and learning processes. An increase or decrease in the number of ionotropic glutamate receptors on a postsynaptic cell may lead to long-term potentiation or long-term depression of that cell, respectively [27–30].

According to Tan et al. [31], there is evidence that reduction in hippocampal glutamate concentrations is associated with improved cognitive function by modulating glutamatergic neurotransmission in non-DS people with AD. Also, murine models of DS suggest that there is an imbalance between hippocampal inhibitory and excitatory inputs [9, 24], changes in the levels of the glutamate transporter and vesicular glutamate transporter 1 (VGLUT1) [25], and impairments in signaling mechanisms downstream of the N-methyl-D-aspartate (NMDA) receptor [26]. In this context, it can be put into consideration that malfunctions in the glutamate metabolism and the glutamatergic system are major contributors to cognitive abnormalities.

In recent studies, it has been shown that patients with DS present a diminution of glutamate and glutamatergic synapses. In the research made with mice by Kaur et al. [32], the results indicated a downregulation of hippocampal glutamate associated with behavioral impairments and intellectual disabilities. In this context, our study aimed to analyze the differential expression of 26 glutamate receptor genes in DS brain samples from prenatal patients to adult age in several brain structures. Overall, our result showed the complexity in the expression of the 26 glutamate receptors encoding genes. Also, a general overexpression in brain samples of GRIN3A and GRIN2C, and higher expression levels of GRM1, GRID2, and GRIK1 in hippocampus, in comparison with some structures of brain cortex. We hypothesize that disruption of glutamatergic brain gene expression would be a crucial early step in the pathogenesis of cognitive disability in DS.

2. Glutamate receptors and DS

Glutamate is known to be the main excitatory neurotransmitter in the brain and under normal physiological conditions, mediates learning and memory, as well as other integrating brain functions of higher order; however, it is also known that the pathological signaling of glutamate contributes to neuronal cell death. This neurotransmitter is released in the synapse after the depolarization of the presynaptic neurons, and it is eliminated by means of the GLT transporter in astrocytes, in normal physiological conditions, glutamate elimination being rapid and neuroprotective [33]. Glutamate has action on ionotropic (iGluR) and metabotropic (mGluRs) receptors. The ionotropic GluRs are ion channels (voltage sensitive), integral membrane proteins composed by four large subunits that form a central ion channel pore [34]. Glutamate receptor subunits are modular structures that contain the following domains: the extracellular amino-terminal domain (ATD), the extracellular ligand-binding domain (LBD), the transmembrane domain (TMD), and an intracellular carboxyl-terminal domain (CTD) [34].

These receptor subunits are proteins assembled into heterotetrameric or homotetrameric receptors, including the N-methyl-D-aspartate receptor (NMDA) consisting of the subunits GluN1, GluN2A, GluN2B, GluN2C, GluN2D, GluN3A, and GluN3B, α-amino-3-hydroxy-5-methyl-4-isoxazolepropionic acid (AMPA) with the subunits GluA1, GluA2, GluA3, and GluA4, and the Kainate receptors with the subunits GluK1, GluK2, GluK3, GluK4, and GluK5 that function as mediators of the rapid synaptic responses to glutamate, contrary to what happens with mGluRs where their activation by glutamate is sensitive to ligand binding and produces slower and longer modulating alterations in synaptic activity [33, 35–37]. NMDA receptors are present in high density within the hippocampus and the cerebral cortex performing fundamental physiological and pathophysiological functions in the central nervous system [38], among which learning, memory, brain plasticity, and recovery of injuries stand out. In these brain structures, differential expression of these receptors is evidenced, where a change in their dynamics could contribute to changes in cognitive and synaptic function [39]. When treated in conjunction with AMPA, they are attributed an important role in plasticity and synaptic transmission in many postsynaptic membranes [35, 40], with the latter receptors participating in protein-protein interactions with scaffolding proteins, such as PICK1 and GRIP1, and the TARP accessory proteins that help in AMPA receptor traffic and present additional targets for regulation [37].

Metabotropic glutamate receptors are members of the superfamily of G protein-coupled receptors. There are eight mGluR subtypes divided into three groups based on sequence homology, G-protein coupling specificity, and pharmacological profile. In general, mGluRs of group I and their interacting proteins have the ability to function as both neuroprotective and neurotoxic and have also been implicated in neurodegenerative diseases, especially mGluR5 [33]. On the other hand, members of group II act by inhibiting neuronal responses in rats according to the studies of Copeland et al. [41], which has been associated with the onset of cognitive deficit, a characteristic that can be observed in people with DS. About this syndrome, it should be noted that it has been associated with an imbalance of excitatory/inhibitory neurotransmitter systems, as highlighted in studies of murine with DS where the presence of alterations in the activity of glutamatergic neurotransmission, mainly affecting ionotropic receptors, an event that has also been evidenced when studying the overexpression of HSA21 genes in DS [42].

3. Glutamatergic system, cognition, and DS: our main approach

The glutamatergic system of the brain is one of the two major amino acid systems, being the GABAergic system the major one. This system is very important for information processing in neuronal networks of the neocortex and hippocampus in particular [43, 44], which is why we decided to analyze not only the brain as a whole, but the hippocampus apart. Also, this brain structure has been studied in several articles related to DS [3, 45–47] because of the significant functional repercussion in memory processes and intellectual potential that follows the poor hippocampal development presented by individuals with DS. Because the glutamatergic system is key in cognition processes such as memory and learning [48, 49], we consider that the deregulation of the glutamate receptors could be critical in the pathophysiology of DS, specifically in the neurodevelopmental and neurocognitive defects. This can be a starting point for developing therapeutic strategies aimed to reduce the effects of altered brain structures in individuals with DS.

3.1 Our methodological approach

Our initial approach was to analyze the expression of glutamate receptors—ionotropic and metabotropic—(**Table A1**) in DS brain samples and compare it to euploid controls. In order to accomplish this goal, we calculated the values of expression for selected genes by using the log10 transformed expression values of a DNA microarray experiment whose registration code and free access in the

GEO database was GSE59630 (http://www.ncbi.nlm.nih.gov/geo/query/acc.cgi?acc=GSE59630), previously deposited by Olmos-Serrano et al. [50], which fitted the statistical significance sample size to obtain trustable information about the functional neurogenomics in DS. The microarray experiment selected included gene expression data of 47,000 probes from 58 postmortem brain samples of DS patients and 58 postmortem brain samples of healthy controls classified by gender (25 from females and 33 from males of each condition), age (from 16 prenatal weeks to 42 years old), and in 11 structures: dorsolateral prefrontal cortex (DFC), visual cortex (V1C), cerebellar cortex (CBC), orbitofrontal cortex (OFC), ventral frontal cortex (VFC), inferior temporal cortex (ITC), hippocampus (HIP), medial frontal cortex (MFC), somatosensory cortex (S1C), inferior parietal cortex (IPC), and superior temporal cortex (STC).

3.2 Functional analysis

The software Cytoscape 3.6 [51] was used for visualizing and analyzing the protein-protein interaction network among the selected human glutamate receptors encoding genes. We use the BIOGrid database to obtain protein interaction data of each one of the genes evaluated. Biological Networks Gene Ontology plugin—BiNGO tool—[52] was used to search in which gene ontology (GO) categories are significantly overrepresented in a set of genes. A hypergeometric test was applied to determine which were the significantly represented categories (p-value <0.05); significant values were adjusted using the Bonferroni family wise error rate correction [53]. From network analyzer plugin of the Max Planck Institute Informatik, network topology parameters were calculated. Moreover, a genetic interaction network was made in GENEMANIA (https://genemania.org/).

3.3 Z-score transformation

Log2 data for each gene in the DNA microarray experiment was log10 transformed and then used for the calculation of Z score [54]. Z scores were calculated by subtracting the mean log gene intensities (within a single experiment) from the log intensity data for each gene, and dividing that result by the SD of all measured log intensities, according to Eq. (1):

Z-score transformation:

$$Z - score = \frac{(Log\ intensity\ of\ G - mean\ \mathrm{log}intensity\ G...Gn)}{Standard\ Deviation\ \mathrm{log}G...Gn} \tag{1}$$

All Z-score values were normalized on a linear scale $-3.0 < 0 > +3.0$. In it, the corresponding gene is overexpressed if the value of Z-score is greater than zero and on contrary is under-expressed if its value is negative.

3.4 Multivariate statistical analysis

Nonparametric analyses for comparing median values of Z-score were performed among gender and age variables between DS patients and healthy control. Wilcoxon signed-rank test was used to calculate the differences between medians of two samples. Hierarchical clustering analysis (HCA) was selected as a method of cluster analysis that seeks to build a hierarchy of clusters [55]. To perform the HCA, Euclidean distance was used as a measure of distance between DS and control samples of Z-score values in several structures of brain cortex; $p < 0.05$ was defined as a threshold. Moreover, principal component analysis (PCA) was employed as a computational procedure for the classification of multiclass gene expression in brain cortex structures between DS and control samples per sex and age. All analyses were run in SPSS program version 22 [56].

4. Our results

4.1 Protein-protein interaction (PPI) network and gene interactions

The PPI network made in Cytoscape 3.6 with all ionotropic and metabotropic receptors had 142 nodes and 3 connected components (**Figure 1**). The proteins encoded by GRIA2 and GRIN2B had the highest amount of interactions (33 and 30, respectively). GRIA2 gene encodes a subunit of the family of glutamate AMPA receptors; these types of receptors mediate fast excitatory synaptic transmission. GRIN2B is also a subunit but, in this case, of a NMDA receptor which are involved in brain development, synaptic plasticity, learning, and memory. The malfunction of these two genes has been previously associated to neurodevelopmental disorders characterized by intellectual disability and delayed development of speech and motor skills [57–59]. Here, it is important to highlight that the many connections they have among the glutamatergic system make them key proteins in the brain protein homeostasis. Among the biological processes ontology categories associated to the network, there was synaptic transmission (P-value Bonferroni 6.44E-17) and transmission of nerve impulse (P-value Bonferroni 1.20E-15).

On the other hand, the gene interaction network made in GENEMANIA showed that the physical interactions with the highest weight are GRIN2A-GRIN1 (9.40E-01), CACNG2-GRIA1 (8.66E-01), and GRIK1-GRIK2 (8.35E-01). The gene GRIN2A encodes a subunit of a subset of NMDA receptors called GluN2A, mainly expressed in regions in the brain involved in speech and language; this gene is consistently referred to in the literature as associated with speech disorders such as impaired intelligibility of

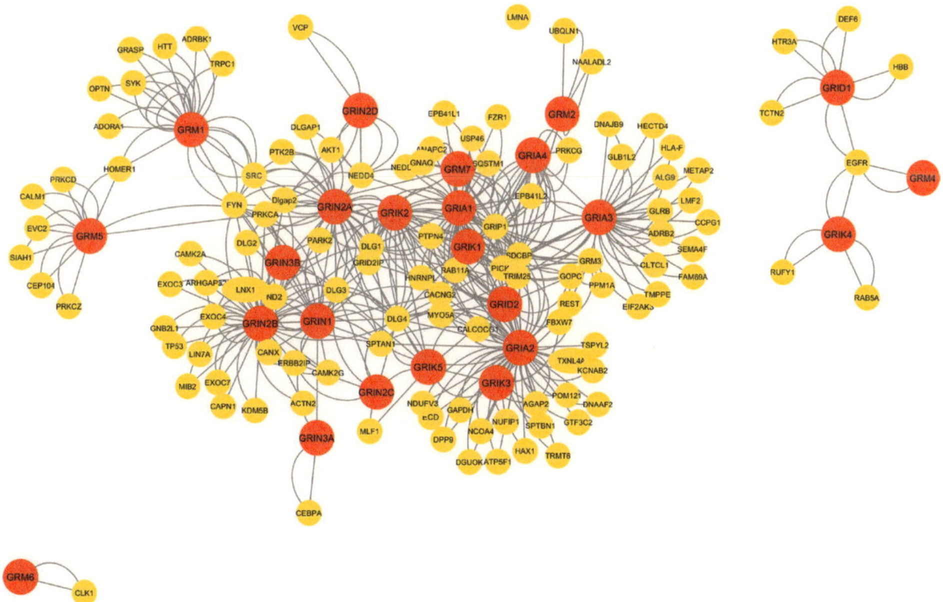

Figure 1.
PPI network made with glutamate receptors in Cytoscape 3.6. The receptors analyzed in this study are shown in red; the interactors are shown in yellow.

conversational speech [60]. GRIN1, on the other hand, also encodes a subunit of NMDA receptors called GluN1, which, along with other members of this superfamily, plays a key role in memory and learning. According to Chen et al. [61], several mutations on this gene have been associated with neurodevelopmental disorders such as epilepsy, causing in some patients hypotonia and facial dysmorphisms. GRIK1 and GRIK2 encode subunits of the kainite family of glutamate receptors, associated with behavior according to the GWAS Catalog (https://www.ebi.ac.uk/gwas/) and with intellectual disability [62].

4.2 Temporal and spatial gene expression in postmortem brains of DS patients

According to the temporal gene expression analysis made, there were no significant differences among the DS brain samples and the control group (**Figure 2**). This is contrasting to the results obtained in other studies focused on mice like the article published by Zhao et al. [63] where they found a difference between older and younger organisms when measuring the expression of glutamate receptors; in their experiment, they found that NMDA receptor functions, receptor subunit composition, and/or the environment in which the receptor interacted were not the same in the old mice as in younger mice which may contribute to the memory decline seen during aging. Also, there is a study made on embryo chicks and 1-year-old chicks by Batista et al. [64] where they found that AMPA receptors exhibit temporal expression changes during tectal development of chicks that are compatible with such a role for glutamate. All the glutamate receptor subunits tested in that experiment—GluR1, GluR2/3, and GluR4—showed an early expression suggesting some function in neurogenesis and migration.

The analysis of gene expression along the different brain structures (**Table 1**) showed an overexpression of the genes Glutamate Ionotropic Receptor NMDA Type Subunit 2C (GRIN2C) (Z-ratio 2.61) and the Glutamate Ionotropic Receptor NMDA Type Subunit 3A (GRIN3A) (2.94). GRIN2C encodes a subunit of an NMDA receptor, which is a subtype of ionotropic glutamate receptor involved in excitatory neurotransmission and in neuronal cell death. On the other hand, GRIN3A also encodes a subunit of a NMDA receptor and its deficit increases spine density and initiates synapse maturation and memory consolidation in early postnatal neurodevelopment; both of these genes have been previously associated with schizophrenia.

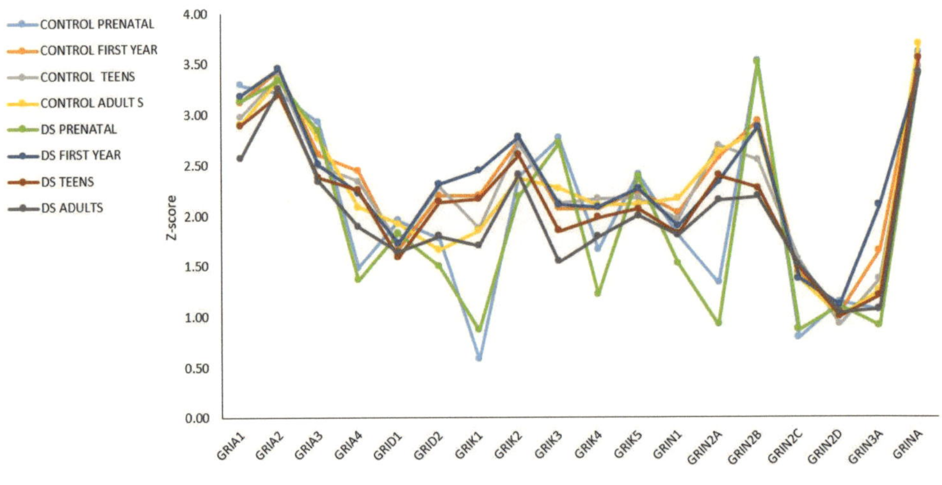

Figure 2.
Z-score of glutamate ionotropic receptors per age-range of control and DS brain samples. Prenatal: 16–22 pregestational weeks, 8 months to 1 year; teens: 12–18 years; and adults: 19–42 years.

Gene symbol	Z-score control	Z-score DS	ΔZ-score	Z ratio*
Ionotropics				
GRIA1	1.88	1.75	−0.12	0.93
GRIA2	2.28	2.21	−0.07	0.97
GRIA3	1.46	1.21	−0.25	0.83
GRIA4	0.97	0.79	−0.18	0.82
GRID1	0.45	0.32	−0.13	0.71
GRID2	0.71	0.76	0.05	1.07
GRIK1	0.58	0.74	0.16	1.28
GRIK2	1.36	1.36	0.00	1.00
GRIK3	0.91	0.59	−0.32	0.65
GRIK4	0.77	0.59	−0.18	0.77
GRIK5	0.91	0.85	−0.05	0.94
GRIN1	0.74	0.49	−0.24	0.67
GRIN2A	1.30	0.92	−0.37	0.71
GRIN2B	1.69	1.32	−0.38	0.78
GRIN2C	0.01	0.02	0.01	2.61
GRIN2D	−0.45	−0.38	0.07	0.85
GRIN3A	0.02	0.07	0.05	2.94
GRINA	2.52	2.36	−0.16	0.94
Metabotropics				
GRM1	0.29	0.20	−0.09	0.69
GRM2	0.27	−0.15	−0.43	−0.57
GRM3	1.66	1.54	−0.13	0.92
GRM4	0.28	0.33	0.06	1.20
GRM5	1.35	1.39	0.05	1.03
GRM6	−0.99	−0.96	0.03	0.97
GRM7	0.48	0.34	−0.15	0.69
GRM8	−0.52	−0.70	0.18	1.34

Log2 data for gene expression were obtained from the microarray experiment consigned in the GEO database with ID GSE59630, previously deposited by Olmos et al.

**Z-Ratio ≥ 1.50 is statistically significant; alpha 0.05.*

Table 1.
Differential expression values (Z-score and Z-ratio) of glutamate receptor encoding genes in the brain of patients with Down syndrome.

According to Ohi et al. [65], GRIN3A expression levels in the dorsolateral prefrontal cortex were elevated by approximately 30% in schizophrenia patients relative to controls, which suggest that aberrant enhanced GRIN3A function could be involved in the pathophysiology of schizophrenia and its cognitive impairments. Another study by Marco et al. [66] in patients with Huntington's disease (HD) and in a mouse model of HD found something similar; a knockout of this gene decreased motor and cognitive dysfunction compared with no knockout and prevented striatal atrophy and synaptic disconnection. These findings correlate with our results of human DS brains, leading us to propose that a similar process might take place in the pathophysiology of DS.

Moreover, we decided to analyze the hippocampus apart because of its highly recognized importance not only in Down syndrome, but also in cognition processes, which are mainly regulated by the glutamatergic system [67]. Several studies have agreed that NMDA receptor (NMDAR)-dependent LTP or an LTP-like process in the hippocampus are the neural substrate for associative spatial learning and memory [68]. In this study, we found that this brain structure has some differences in gene expression when compared to the brain as a whole. While the general analysis of the brain showed an overexpression of the gene GRIN3A, at the hippocampus, we encountered an under-expression if this gene in DS samples. On the other hand, a gene that encodes the Glutamate

Gene symbol	Z-score control	Z-score DS	ΔZ-score	Z ratio*
Ionotropics				
GRIA1	2.15	2.25	0.10	1.04
GRIA2	2.48	2.35	−0.13	0.95
GRIA3	1.59	1.62	0.03	1.02
GRIA4	0.14	−0.07	−0.21	−0.49
GRID1	0.59	0.55	−0.04	0.93
GRID2	0.18	0.47	0.29	2.61
GRIK1	0.37	0.60	0.23	1.62
GRIK2	1.35	1.20	0.15	0.88
GRIK3	0.58	−0.19	−0.77	−0.32
GRIK4	0.96	0.95	−0.01	0.99
GRIK5	1.14	1.22	0.08	1.07
GRIN1	0.74	0.49	−0.25	0.67
GRIN2A	1.28	1.15	−0.13	0.90
GRIN2B	1.74	1.73	−0.01	0.99
GRIN2C	0.19	0.34	0.15	1.85
GRIN2D	−0.56	−0.41	0.15	0.73
GRIN3A	0.35	−0.22	−0.57	−0.62
GRINA	2.40	2.28	−0.12	0.95
Metabotropics				
GRM1	0.10	0.22	0.12	2.22
GRM2	0.10	−0.54	−0.64	−5.62
GRM3	1.68	1.30	−0.38	0.77
GRM4	0.12	0.05	−0.07	0.44
GRM5	1.51	1.62	0.11	1.07
GRM6	−0.96	−0.87	0.09	0.91
GRM7	0.71	0.51	−1.22	0.72
GRM8	−0.54	−0.75	−0.21	1.37

Log2 data for gene expression were obtained from the microarray experiment consigned in the GEO database with ID GSE59630, previously deposited by Olmos et al.

**Z-Ratio ≥ 1.50 is statistically significant; alpha 0.05.*

Table 2.
Differential expression values of glutamate receptor encoding genes in the hippocampus of patients with Down syndrome.

Metabotropic Receptor 1 (GRM1) was overexpressed in the hippocampus (Z-ratio 2.22) as well as the Glutamate Ionotropic Receptor Delta Type Subunit 2 (GRID2) (Z-score 2.61), the Glutamate Ionotropic Receptor Kainate Type Subunit 1 (GRIK1) (Z-score 1.62), and GRIN2C (Z-score 1.85). GRM1 is one of the most abundant mGluRs in the mammalian central nervous system and is present at particularly high levels in Purkinje cells [69]. There is plenty of evidence of its implication in diseases involving glutamatergic dysfunction and abnormal synaptic plasticity [70], which are known to be crucial mechanisms for cognitive processes. GRIK1 has also been reported as overexpressed in studies of DS; the study made on mice by Mazier [71] showed that GRIK mRNA levels are increased by more than 50% in different structures of the trisomic brain, which is coincidental with our findings (**Table 2**).

4.3 Principal component analysis (PCA) and hierarchical cluster analysis (HCA)

According to the PCA performed for the control samples, five principal components explained 80% of the cumulative variance; meanwhile, the PCA performed for the DS samples showed that six principal components explained 83% of the cumulative variance. In **Figure 3**, we present the PCA for the two groups, where we found some differences in the clustering of genes when comparing the group samples, specifically in genes GRID2, GRM1, GRM4, and GRIK2 which were closely grouped in the PCA for controls. Also, even though the gene GRIK1 remained on the same position in both PCA, its association with GRIA1 changed from being separated in the control group, to be near each other in the DS group.

The HCA analysis produced a Heatmap that showed gene expression differences in the hippocampus (**Figure 4**), specifically in the genes Glutamate Ionotropic Receptor Kainate Type Subunit 3 (GRIK3) and GRIN3A which were under-expressed in DS samples as mentioned previously. GRIK3 has not been related to DS in particular, but it has been widely studied for its association with schizophrenia and major depression [72, 73]. Overall, the expression of the glutamate metabotropic receptors was especially high in the OFC in comparison to other brain structures.

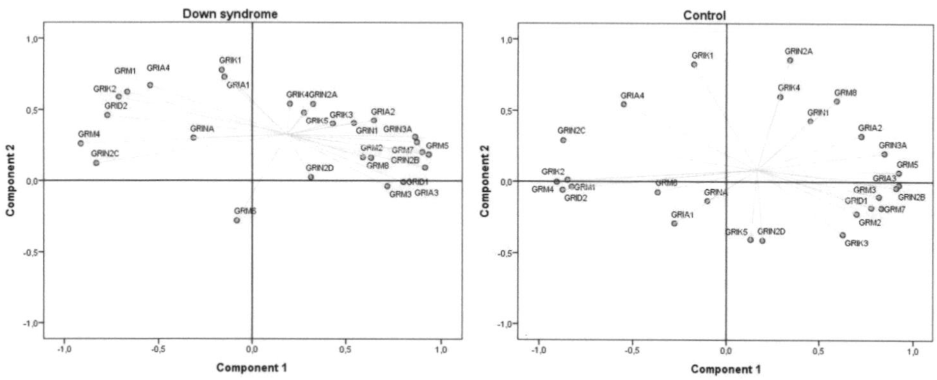

Figure 3.
Principal component analysis in 11 brain structures in DS brain samples and controls: dorsolateral prefrontal cortex (DFC), visual cortex (V1C), cerebellar cortex (CBC), orbitofrontal cortex (OFC), ventral frontal cortex (VFC), inferior temporal cortex (ITC), hippocampus (HIP), medial frontal cortex (MFC), somatosensory cortex (S1C), inferior parietal cortex (IPC), and superior temporal cortex (STC). Analyses were performed in SPSS v 22.0.

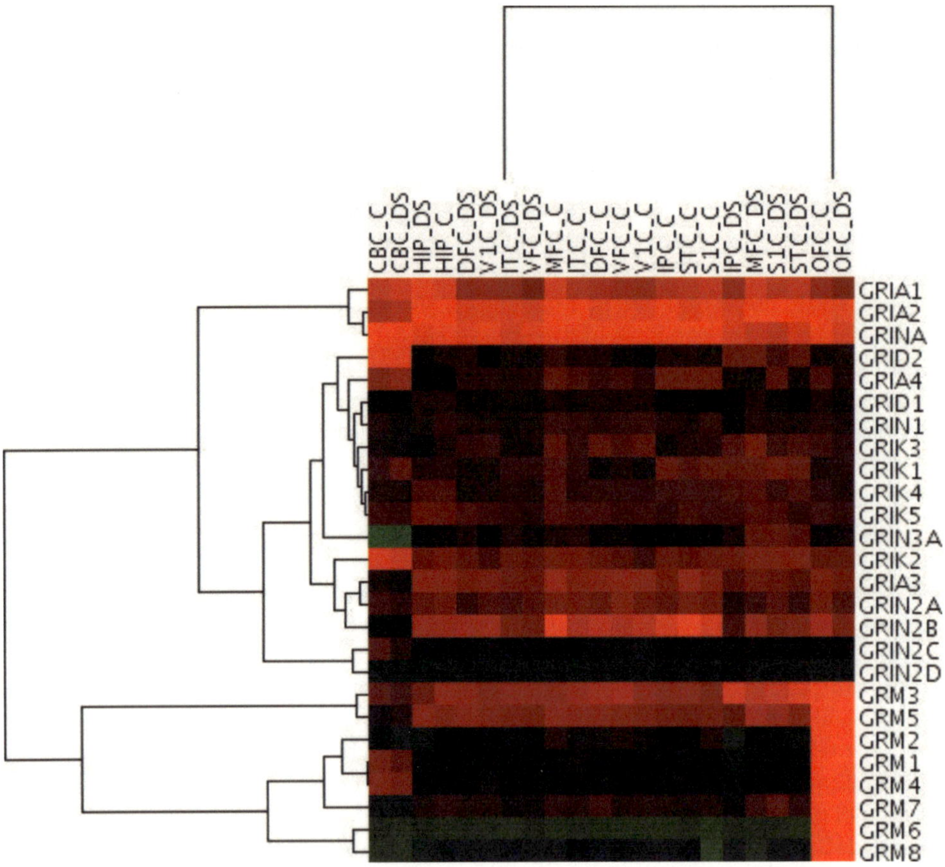

Figure 4.
Heat map of glutamate receptor expression of 11 brain structures in DS brain samples and controls. Green color represents under-expression and red overexpression: dorsolateral prefrontal cortex (DFC), visual cortex (V1C), cerebellar cortex (CBC), orbitofrontal cortex (OFC), ventral frontal cortex (VFC), inferior temporal cortex (ITC), hippocampus (HIP), medial frontal cortex (MFC), somatosensory cortex (S1C), inferior parietal cortex (IPC), and superior temporal cortex (STC); performed in Cytoscape 3.6 software.

5. Conclusions

The glutamatergic system is closely related to cognition as it plays a key role in memory, working memory, and executive functions. It has been proven in mice with DS that a deregulation of this system can be crucial in both the neurodevelopmental and neurodegenerative components of DS. DS patients have intellectual disabilities with individual variability in the severity of both physiological and behavioral phenotypes. At the core of the intellectual disabilities is the phenomenon of synaptic plasticity, which is a functional change in the strength at the points of communication between neurons. Our results indicate hippocampal downregulation of the ionotropic receptor subunit GRIN3A (NMDA family), while in the general analysis of the brain, this gene was overexpressed. Other genes overexpressed in the hippocampus were the metabotropic receptor GRM1, the ionotropic receptor subunit GRID2, and the kainate receptor subunit GRIK1. This deregulation might produce an alteration of both presynaptic and postsynaptic dysfunction at glutamatergic synapses, possibly contributing to behavioral impairments in patients with DS.

In general, our results suggest the existence of a fine regulation mechanism of gene expression networks, which is involved in the glutamatergic synaptic system in several structures of brain from patients with DS. We hypothesize that disruption of glutamatergic brain gene expression would be a crucial early step in the pathogenesis of cognitive disability in DS. Moreover, our results suggest that glutamatergic system in association with other neurotransmitter systems in human brain, as GABA-mediated synaptic inhibition reported in other DS studies, might associate with glutamatergic receptor alterations to bring upon synaptic changes and cognitive deficits in DS models. Thus, glutamatergic receptor gene expression dysfunction may play a key role in the hippocampal pathogenesis of DS.

Acknowledgements

The authors are grateful to the Universidad del Valle for the financing of some of the projects executed by LABIOMOL research group at the Department of the Physiological Sciences, School of Basic Sciences of the Faculty of Health, Universidad del Valle in Cali, Colombia. Within the document, the corresponding credits are given to both freely accessible bioinformatic platforms and the different computational tools used in the execution of the present study.

Conflict of interest

On behalf of all authors, the corresponding author states that there is no conflict of interest.

Supplementary information

ID	Gene symbol	Subunit	Official full name	Locus
		Ionotropic family		
2890	GRIA1	GluA1 ($GluR_1$)	Glutamate ionotropic receptor AMPA type subunit 1	5q33.2
2891	GRIA2	GluA2 ($GluR_2$)	Glutamate ionotropic receptor AMPA type subunit 2	4q32.1
2892	GRIA3	GluA3 ($GluR_3$)	Glutamate ionotropic receptor AMPA type subunit 3	Xq25
2893	GRIA4	GluA4 ($GluR_4$)	Glutamate ionotropic receptor AMPA type subunit 4	11q22.3
2894	GRID1	GluD1 (GluRD1)	Glutamate ionotropic receptor delta type subunit 1	10q23.1-q23.2
2895	GRID2	GluD2 (GlurD2)	Glutamate ionotropic receptor delta type subunit 2	4q22.1-q22.2
		Kainate family		
2897	GRIK1	GluK1 ($GluR_5$)	Glutamate ionotropic receptor kainate type subunit 1	21q21.3
2898	GRIK2	GluK2 ($GluR_6$)	Glutamate ionotropic receptor kainate type subunit 2	6q16.3
2899	GRIK3	GluK3 ($GluR_7$)	Glutamate ionotropic receptor kainate type subunit 3	1p34.3

ID	Gene symbol	Subunit	Official full name	Locus
2900	GRIK4	GluK4 (KA-1)	Glutamate ionotropic receptor kainate type subunit 4	11q23.3
2901	GRIK5	GluK5 (KA-2)	Glutamate ionotropic receptor kainate type subunit 5	19q13.2
		NMDA family		
2902	GRIN1	GluN1(NR1)	Glutamate ionotropic receptor NMDA type subunit 1	9q34.3
2903	GRIN2A	GluN2A (NR2A)	Glutamate ionotropic receptor NMDA type subunit 2A	16p13.2
2904	GRIN2B	GluN2B (NR2B)	Glutamate ionotropic receptor NMDA type subunit 2B	12p13.1
2905	GRIN2C	GluN2C (NR2C)	Glutamate ionotropic receptor NMDA type subunit 2C	17q25.1
2906	GRIN2D	GluN2D (NR2D)	Glutamate ionotropic receptor NMDA type subunit 2D	19q13.33
116,443	GRIN3A	GluN3A (NR3A)	Glutamate ionotropic receptor NMDA type subunit 3A	9q31.1
2907	GRINA	GluN3B (NR3B)	Glutamate ionotropic receptor NMDA type subunit associated protein 1	8q24.3
Metabotropic family group 1				
2911	GRM1	mGluR$_1$	Glutamate metabotropic receptor 1	6q24.3
2915	GRM5	mGluR$_4$	Glutamate metabotropic receptor 5	11q14.2-q14.3
Metabotropic family group 2				
2912	GRM2	mGluR$_5$	Glutamate metabotropic receptor 2	3p21.2
2913	GRM3	mGluR$_2$	Glutamate metabotropic receptor 3	7q21.11-q21.12
Metabotropic family group 3				
2914	GRM4	mGluR$_3$	Glutamate metabotropic receptor 4	6p21.31
2916	GRM6	mGluR$_6$	Glutamate metabotropic receptor 6	5q35.3
2917	GRM7	mGluR$_7$	Glutamate metabotropic receptor 7	3p26.1
2918	GRM8	mGluR$_8$	Glutamate metabotropic receptor 8	7q31.33

Information taken from the NCBI—Genbank platform.

Table A1.
Description of glutamate receptors encoding genes.

Author details

Alejandra Rocio Rodríguez Ortiz, Mailyn Alejandra Bedoya Saldarriaga, Julio César Montoya Villegas and Felipe García-Vallejo*
Investigation group LABIOMOL, Universidad del Valle, Cali, Colombia

*Address all correspondence to: labiomol@gmail.com

References

[1] Nadel L. Down's syndrome: A genetic disorder in biobehavioral perspective. Genes, Brain, and Behavior. 2003;**2**:156-166. DOI: 10.1034/j.1601-183x.2003.00026.x

[2] Antonarakis ES, Epstein CJ. The challenge of Down syndrome. Trends in Molecular Medicine. 2006;**12**:473-479. DOI: 10.1016/j.molmed.2006.08.005

[3] Sylvester PE. The hippocampus in Down's syndrome. Journal of Mental Deficiency Research. 1983;**27**(Pt 3): 227-236. DOI: 10.1111/j.1365-2788.1983.tb00294.x

[4] Coyle JT, Oster-Granite ML, Gearhart JD. The neurobiology consequences of Down syndrome. Brain Research Bulletin. 1986;**16**:773-787. DOI: 10.1016/0361-9230(86)90074-2

[5] Shapiro BL. Developmental instability of the cerebellum and its relevance to Down syndrome. Journal of Neural Transmission. Supplementum. 2001;**61**:11-34. DOI: 10.1007/978-3-7091-6262-0_2

[6] Larsen KB, Laursen H, Græmb N, Samuelsena GB, Bogdanovicc N, Pakkenberga B. Reduced cell number in the neocortical part of the human fetal brain in Down syndrome. Annals of Anatomy. 2008;**190**:421-427. DOI: 10.1016/j.aanat.2008.05.007

[7] Contestabile A, Fila T, Ceccarelli C, Bonasone P, Bonapace L, Santini D, et al. Cell cycle alteration and decreased cell proliferation in the hippocampal dentate gyrus and in the neocortical germinal matrix of fetuses with Down syndrome and in Ts65Dn mice. Hippocampus. 2007;**17**:665-678. DOI: 10.1002/hipo.20308

[8] Vicari S. Memory development and intellectual disabilities. Acta Paediatrica. 2004;(Suppl 93):60-63. DOI: 10.1111/j.1651-2227.2004.tb03059.x

[9] Vicari S, Bellucci S, Carlesimo GA. Implicit and explicit memory: A functional dissociation in persons with Down syndrome. Neuropsychologia. 2000;**38**:240-251. DOI: 10.1016/s0028-3932(99)00081-0

[10] Vicari S, Bellucci S, Carlesimo GA. Visual and spatial long-term memory: Differential pattern of impairments in Williams and Down syndromes. Developmental Medicine and Child Neurology. 2005;**47**:305-311. DOI: 10.1017/s0012162205000599

[11] Vicari S, Pontillo M, Armando M. Neurodevelopmental and psychiatric issues in Down's syndrome: Assessment and intervention. Psychiatric Genetics. 2013;**23**:95-107. DOI: 10.1097/YPG.0b013e32835fe426

[12] Hyman BT, West HL, Rebeck GW, Lai F, Mann DMA. Neuropathological changes in Down's syndrome hippocampal formation effect of age and apolipoprotein E genotype. Archives of Neurology. 1995;**52**(4):373-378. DOI: 10.1001/archneur.1995.00540280059019

[13] Teipel SJ, Hampel H. Neuroanatomy of Down syndrome in vivo: A model of preclinical Alzheimer's disease. Behavior Genetics. 2006;**36**(3):405-401. DOI: 10.1007/s10519-006-9047-x

[14] Brassai A, Suvanjeiev RG, Bán EG, Lakatos M. Role of synaptic and nonsynaptic glutamate receptors in ischaemia induced neurotoxicity. Review. Brain Research Bulletin. 2015;**112**:1-6. DOI: 10.1016/j.brainresbull.2014.12.007

[15] Petroff OA. GABA and glutamate in the human brain. The Neuroscientist. 2002;**8**(6):562-573. DOI: 10.1177/1073858402238515

[16] Watanabe M, Maemura K, Kanbara K, Tamayama T, Hayasaki H. GABA and

GABA receptors in the central nervous system and other organs. International Review of Cytology. 2002;**213**:1-47. DOI: 10.1016/S0074-7696(02)13011-7

[17] Reiner A, Levitz J. Glutamatergic signaling in the central nervous system: Ionotropic and metabotropic receptors in concert. Neuron. 2018;**98**(6):1080-1098. DOI: 10.1016/j.neuron.2018.05.018

[18] Debanne D, Daoudal G, Sourdet V, Russier M. Brain plasticity and ion channels. Journal of Physiology, Paris. 2003;**97**(4-6):403-414. DOI: 10.1016/j.jphysparis.2004.01.004

[19] Maren S, Tocco G, Standley S, Baudry M, Thompson RF. Postsynaptic factors in the expression of long-term potentiation (LTP): Increased glutamate receptor binding following LTP induction in vivo. PNAS. 1993;**90**(20):9654-9658. DOI: 10.1073/pnas.90.20.9654

[20] Pérez-Otaño I, Ehlers MD. Homeostatic plasticity and NMDA receptor trafficking. Trends in Neurosciences. 2005;**28**(5):229-238. DOI: 10.1016/j.tins.2005.03.004

[21] Asztély F, Gustafsson B. Ionotropic glutamate receptors. Their possible role in the expression of hippocampal synaptic plasticity. Molecular Neurobiology. 1996;**12**(1):1-11. DOI: 10.1007/BF02740744

[22] Weiler IJ, Greenough WT. Metabotropic glutamate receptors trigger postsynaptic protein synthesis. PNAS. 1993;**90**(15):7168-7171. DOI: 10.1073/pnas.90.15.7168

[23] Teichberg VI. Glial glutamate receptors: Likely actors in brain signaling. The FASEB Journal. 1991;**5**(15):3086-3091. DOI: 10.1096/fasebj.5.15.1660422

[24] Steinhäuser C, Gallo V. News on glutamate receptors in glial cells. Trends in Neurosciences. 1996;**19**(8):339-345. DOI: 10.1016/0166-2236(96)10043-6

[25] Ohashi H, Maruyama T, Higashi-Matsumoto H, Nomoto T, Nishimura S, Takeuchi Y. A novel binding assay for metabotropic glutamate receptors using [3H] L-quisqualic acid and recombinant receptors. Zeitschrift für Naturforschung. 2002;**57**(3-4):348-355. DOI: 10.1515/znc-2002-3-425

[26] Soares C, Lee KF, Nassrallah W, Béïque JC. Differential subcellular targeting of glutamate receptor subtypes during homeostatic synaptic plasticity. The Journal of Neuroscience. 2013;**33**(33):13547-13559. DOI: 10.1523/JNEUROSCI.1873-13.2013

[27] Adesnik H, Nicoll RA. Conservation of glutamate receptor 2-containing AMPA receptors during long-term potentiation. The Journal of Neuroscience. 2007;**27**:4598-4602. DOI: 10.1523/JNEUROSCI.0325-07.2007

[28] Henley JM, Wilkinson KA. AMPA receptor trafficking and the mechanisms underlying synaptic plasticity and cognitive aging. Dialogues in Clinical Neuroscience. 2013;**15**(1):11-27

[29] Bliss T, Collingridge G. A synaptic model of memory: Long-term potentiation in the hippocampus. Nature. 1993;**361**:31-39. DOI: 10.1038/361031a0

[30] Murugan M, Ling EA, Kaur C. Glutamate receptors in microglia. CNS & Neurological Disorders Drug Targets. 2013;**12**(6):773-784. DOI: 10.2174/18715273113126660174

[31] Tan GM, Beacher F, Daly E, Horder J, Prasher V, Hanney ML, et al. Hippocampal glutamate-glutamine (Glx) in adults with Down syndrome: A preliminary study using in vivo proton magnetic resonance spectroscopy ((1)H MRS). Journal of Neurodevelopmental

Disorders. 2014;**6**(1):42. DOI: 10.1186/1866-1955-6-42

[32] Kaur G, Sharma A, Xu W, Gerum S, Alldred MJ, Subbanna S, et al. Glutamatergic transmission aberration: A major cause of behavioral deficits in a murine model of Down's syndrome. The Journal of Neuroscience. 2014;**34**(15):5099-5106. DOI: 10.1523/JNEUROSCI.5338-13.2014

[33] Hamilton A, Zamponi GW, Ferguson SS. Glutamate receptors function as scaffolds for the regulation of β-amyloid and cellular prion protein signaling complexes. Molecular Brain. 2015;**8**:18. DOI: 10.1186/s13041-015-0107-0

[34] Traynelis SF, Wollmuth LP, Mcbain CJ, Menniti FS, Vance KM, Ogden KK, et al. Glutamate receptor ion channels: Structure, regulation, and function. Pharmacological Reviews. 2010;**62**(3):405-496. DOI: 10.1124/pr.109.002451

[35] Hamilton A, Esseltine JL, Devries RA, Cregan SP, Ferguson SSG. Metabotropic glutamate receptor 5 knockout reduces cognitive impairment and pathogenesis in a mouse model of Alzheimer's disease. Molecular Brain. 2014;**7**:40. DOI: 10.1186/1756-6606-7-40

[36] Regan MC, Furukawa H. Previews deeper insights into the allosteric modulation of ionotropic glutamate receptors. Neuron. 2016;**91**(6):1187-1189. DOI: 10.1016/j.neuron.2016.09.013

[37] Rojas A, Dingledine R. Ionotropic glutamate receptors: Regulation by G-protein-coupled receptors. Molecular Pharmacology. 2013;**83**(4):746-752. DOI: 10.1124/mol.112.083352

[38] Samardzic J, Jadzic D, Hencic B. Introductory Chapter: GABA/Glutamate Balance: A Key for Normal Brain Functioning. In: Samardzic J, editor. GABA And Glutamate, New Developments In Neurotransmission Research. London, United Kingdom: IntechOpen; 2018. pp. 1-8. Chapter 1. Available from: https://www.intechopen.com/books/gaba-and-glutamate-new-developments-in-neurotransmission-research/introductory-chapter-gaba-glutamate-balance-a-key-for-normal-brain-functioning

[39] Kumar A. NMDA receptor function during senescence: Implication on cognitive performance. Frontiers in Neuroscience. 2015;**9**:473. DOI: 10.3389/fnins.2015.00473

[40] Sangeeta P, Swapnil S, Sarvesh P, SB K. Receptors involved in learning and memory process. Pharmacology Online. 2017;**3**:7-13

[41] Copeland CS, Neale SA, Salt TE. Neuronal activity patterns in the mediodorsal thalamus and related cognitive circuits are modulated by metabotropic glutamate receptors. Neuropharmacology. 2015;**92**:16-24. DOI: 10.1016/j.neuropharm.2014.12.031

[42] Saud K, Arriagada C, Cárdenas AM, Shimahara T, Allen DD, Caviedes R, et al. Neuronal dysfunction in Down syndrome: Contribution of neuronal models in cell culture. Journal of Physiology, Paris. 2006;**99**(2-3):201-210

[43] Tamminga CA, Southcott S, Sacco C, Wagner AD, Ghose S. Glutamate dysfunction in hippocampus: Relevance of dentate gyrus and CA3 signaling. Schizophrenia Bulletin. 2012;**38**(5):927-935. DOI: 10.1093/schbul/sbs062

[44] Institute of Medicine (US) Forum on Neuroscience and Nervous System Disorders. Overview of the glutamatergic system. In: Glutamate-Related Biomarkers in Drug Development for Disorders of the Nervous System: Workshop Summary. Washington (DC): National Academies

Press (US); 2011. Available from: https://www.ncbi.nlm.nih.gov/books/NBK62187/

[45] Powers BE, Santiago NA, Strupp BJ. Rapid forgetting of social learning in the Ts65Dn mouse model of Down syndrome: New evidence for hippocampal dysfunction. Behavioral Neuroscience. 2018;**132**(1):51-56. DOI: 10.1037/bne0000227

[46] Gómez de Salazar M, Grau C, Ciruela F, Altafaj X. Phosphoproteomic alterations of ionotropic glutamate receptors in the hippocampus of the Ts65Dn mouse model of Down syndrome. Frontiers in Molecular Neuroscience. 2018;**11**:226. DOI: 10.3389/fnmol.2018.00226

[47] Milenkovic I, Stojanovic T, Aronica E, Fülöp L, Bozsó Z, Máté Z, et al. GABAA receptor subunit deregulation in the hippocampus of human fetuses with Down syndrome. Brain Structure & Function. 2018;**223**. DOI: 1501. DOI: 10.1007/s00429-017-1563-3

[48] Peng S, Zhang Y, Zhang J, Wang H, Ren B. Glutamate receptors and signal transduction in learning and memory. Molecular Biology Reports. 2011;**38**(1):453-460. DOI: 10.1007/s11033-010-0128-9

[49] Rezvani AH. Involvement of the NMDA system in learning and memory. In: Levin ED, Buccafusco JJ, editors. Animal Models of Cognitive Impairment. Boca Raton (FL): CRC Press/Taylor & Francis; 2006. Chapter 4. Available from: https://www.ncbi.nlm.nih.gov/books/NBK2532/

[50] Olmos-Serrano JL, Kang HJ, Tyler WA, Silbereis JC, Cheng F, Zhu Y, et al. Down syndrome developmental brain transcriptome reveals defective oligodendrocyte differentiation and myelination. Neuron. 2016;**89**(6):1208-1222. DOI: 10.1016/j.neuron.2016.01.042

[51] Shannon P, Markiel A, Ozier O, Baliga NS, Wang JT, Ramage D, et al. Cytoscape: A software environment for integrated models of biomolecular interaction networks. Genome Research. 2003;**13**(11):2498-2504. DOI: 10.1101/gr.1239303

[52] Maere S, Heymans K, Kuiper M. BiNGO: A Cytoscape plugin to assess overrepresentation of gene ontology categories in biological networks. Bioinformatics. 2005;**21**(16):3448-3449. DOI: 10.1093/bioinformatics/bti551

[53] Armstrong RA. When to use the Bonferroni correction. Ophthalmic & Physiological Optics. 2014;**34**(5):502-508. DOI: 10.1111/opo.12131

[54] Cheadle C, Vawter MP, Freed WJ, Becker KG. Analysis of microarray data using Z Score transformation. The Journal of Molecular Diagnostics. 2003;**5**(2):73-81. DOI: 10.1016/S1525-1578(10)60455-2

[55] Cameron DA, Middleton FA, Chenn A, Olson EC. Hierarchical clustering of gene expression patterns in the Eomes+lineage of excitatory neurons during early neocortical development. BMC Neuroscience. 2012;**13**:90. DOI: 10.1186/1471-2202-13-90

[56] Bicciato S, Luchini A, Di Bello C. PCA disjoint models for multiclass cancer analysis using gene expression data. Bioinformatics. 2003;**19**:571-578

[57] Hu C, Chen W, Myers SJ, Yuan H, Traynelis SF. Human GRIN2B variants in neurodevelopmental disorders. Journal of Pharmacological Sciences. 2016;**132**(2):115-121. DOI: 10.1016/j.jphs.2016.10.002

[58] Platzer K, Lemke JR. GRIN2B-related neurodevelopmental disorder. In: Adam MP, Ardinger HH, Pagon RA, et al., editors. GeneReviews® [Internet]. Seattle (WA): University of Washington, Seattle; 1993-2018.

Available from: https://www.ncbi.nlm.nih.gov/books/NBK501979/ [May 31, 2018]

[59] Soto D, Altafaj X, Sindreu C, Bayés A. Glutamate receptor mutations in psychiatric and neurodevelopmental disorders. Communicative & Integrative Biology. 2014;7(1):e27887. DOI: 10.4161/cib.27887

[60] Myers KA, Scheffer IE. GRIN2A-related speech disorders and epilepsy. In: Adam MP, Ardinger HH, Pagon RA, et al., editors. GeneReviews® [Internet]. Seattle (WA): University of Washington, Seattle; 1993-2018. Available from: https://www.ncbi.nlm.nih.gov/books/NBK385627/ [September 29, 2016]

[61] Chen W, Shieh C, Swanger SA, Tankovic A, Au M, McGuire M, et al. GRIN1 mutation associated with intellectual disability alters NMDA receptor trafficking and function. Journal of Human Genetics. 2017;**62**(6):589-597. DOI: 10.1038/jhg.2017.19

[62] Córdoba M, Rodriguez S, González Morón D, Medina N, Kauffman MA. Expanding the spectrum of Grik2 mutations: Intellectual disability, behavioural disorder, epilepsy and dystonia. Clinical Genetics. 2015;**87**(3):293-295. DOI: 10.1111/cge.12423

[63] Zhao X, Rosenke R, Kronemann D, Brim B, Das SR, Dunah AW, et al. The effects of aging on N-methyl-D-aspartate receptor subunits in the synaptic membrane and relationships to long-term spatial memory. Neuroscience. 2009;**162**(4):933-945. DOI: 10.1016/j.neuroscience.2009.05.018

[64] Batista SS, Pires RS, Britto LRG. Differential expression of AMPA-type glutamate receptor subunits during development of the chick optic tectum. Brazilian Journal of Medical and Biological Research. 2002;**35**(8):973-978. DOI: 10.1590/S0100-879X2002000800015

[65] Ohi K, Hashimoto R, Ikeda M, Yamamori H, Yasuda Y, Fujimoto M, et al. Glutamate networks implicate cognitive impairments in schizophrenia: Genome-wide association studies of 52 cognitive phenotypes. Schizophrenia Bulletin. 2014;**41**(4):909-918. DOI: 10.1093/schbul/sbu171

[66] Marco S, Giralt A, Petrovic MM, Pouladi MA, Martínez-Turrillas R, Martínez-Hernández J, et al. Suppressing aberrant GluN3A expression rescues synaptic and behavioral impairments in Huntington's disease models. Nature Medicine. 2013;**19**:1030-1038. DOI: 10.1038/nm.3246

[67] Cammarota M, Bevilaqua LR, Bonini JS, Rossatto JI, Medina JH, Izquierdo N. Hippocampal glutamate receptors in fear memory consolidation. Neurotoxicity Research. 2004;**6**(3):205-212

[68] Taylor AM, Bus T, Sprengel R, Seeburg PH, Rawlins JN, Bannerman DM. Hippocampal NMDA receptors are important for behavioural inhibition but not for encoding associative spatial memories. Philosophical Transactions of the Royal Society of London. Series B, Biological Sciences. 2014;**369**(1633):20130149. DOI: 10.1098/rstb.2013.0149

[69] Watson LM, Bamber E, Schnekenberg RP, Williams J, Bettencourt C, Lickiss J. Dominant mutations in GRM1 cause spinocerebellar ataxia type 44. American Journal of Human Genetics. 2017;**101**(3):451-458. DOI: 10.1016/j.ajhg.2017.08.005

[70] Power EM, English NA, Empson RM. Are Type 1 metabotropic glutamate

receptors a viable therapeutic target for the treatment of cerebellar ataxia? The Journal of Physiology. 2016;**594**: 4643-4652. DOI: 10.1113/JP271153

[71] Mazier W. Assessing the action of GluK1 overexpression on synaptic strength and plasticity in a mouse model of Down syndrome [Thesis]. Spain: Neuroscience Institute of Alicante, Universidad Miguel Hernandez; 2014

[72] Kilic G, Ismail Kucukali C, Orhan N, Ozkok E, Zengin A, Aydin M, et al. Are GRIK3 (T928G) gene variants in schizophrenia patients different from those in their first-degree relatives? Psychiatry Research. 2010;**175**:43-46. DOI: 10.1016/j.psychres.2008.10.001

[73] Schiffer HH, Heinemann SF. Association of the human kainite receptor GluR7 gene (GRIK3) with recurrent major depressive disorder. American Journal of Medical Genetics. Part B, Neuropsychiatric Genetics. 2007;**144B**:20-26. DOI: 10.1002/ajmg.b.30374

Chapter 3

Gene Activation by the Cytokine-Driven Transcription Factor STAT1

Roswitha Nast, Julia Staab and Thomas Meyer

Abstract

Signal transducers and activators of transcription (STATs) are a family of cytokine-regulated transcription factors, which serve the dual role of external signal transduction and transcriptional activation. The founding member of this family, STAT1, is involved in a plethora of cellular processes, including interferon-dependent upregulation of various effector mechanisms in immune and non-immune cells to control bacterial, fungal and parasitic infections. In this chapter, we discuss the principles of STAT1-driven gene expression and focus on the clinical phenotypes of various human STAT1 mutations. In particular, we highlight the significance of sequence-specific DNA binding and intact nucleocytoplasmic shuttling for full transcriptional activation of interferon-driven target genes.

Keywords: signal transducer and activator of transcription (STAT), Janus kinase (JAK), DNA binding, cytokine signalling, gene expression, interferon, gain-of-function mutation

1. Introduction

The origins of the seminal discovery of the intracellular signal transmitters mediating cytokine signalling now date back nearly three decades. In the late 1980s, a group of researchers observed that signal transmission could be induced within minutes after stimulating cells with type I interferons (IFNs). Such speed, with which the signal generated at the plasma membrane-bound receptor was transduced to the nucleus, suggested the presence of only a few intermediate steps. Eventually, the only two players involved were identified, which are receptor-associated Janus kinases (JAKs) and the signal transducers and activators of transcription (STATs) [1]. The STAT proteins comprise a family of evolutionary highly conserved transcription factors, which are thought to have evolved with the development of the first multicellular organisms [2, 3]. They are expressed in various metazoan animal species, including nematodes, insects and vertebrates [4–9]. In mammals, seven different STAT proteins have been identified, namely STAT1, STAT2, STAT3, STAT4, STAT5A, STAT5B and STAT6. The STATs are differentially activated by a variety of almost 50 extracellular signalling molecules, including interferons, interleukins, growth factors and hormones [10] and are involved in a plethora of biological processes, including cell differentiation, proliferation, development, immunity and apoptosis [11]. STAT1, the founding member of this family, is the major signalling molecule activated by IFN-α/β and IFN-γ and plays a pivotal role in mediating immune responses to infectious pathogens. It is essential for the direct activation of various immune effector genes, including those coding for microbicidal molecules, antiviral proteins, antigen-presenting molecules, phagocytic receptors, chemokines and cytokines [12]. Not surprisingly, humans expressing STAT1 variants with nonsense or missense mutations often exhibit an increased susceptibility to bacterial and viral infections.

2. Design principles of the JAK/STAT signalling pathway

STAT signalling is a paradigm of a ligand-induced pathway from cell surface receptors to the transcriptional machinery, thereby connecting extracellular signals to the regulation of eukaryotic gene expression. The activation of STAT proteins and their mechanisms of action are unique in many ways: (i) This pathway represents one of the first examples of direct signalling to the nucleus without the involvement of second messengers, (ii) post-transcriptional modification by tyrosine phosphorylation is a hallmark feature of this pathway and, (iii) STATs make direct contacts with both membrane-bound receptors and DNA, thereby integrating cellular processes at the membrane to nuclear events. The basic model of STAT signalling depends on a cascade of tyrosine phosphorylation steps, as shown in **Figure 1** [11]. Binding of the ligand to its cognate cell surface receptor triggers the dimerization or multimerization of the transmembrane receptor subunits. Conformational changes in the receptor complex bring the non-covalently attached Janus kinases (JAKs) into close spatial proximity to each other and allow their trans-phosphorylation on specific tyrosine residues. As a result, the JAKs are activated and, in turn, phosphorylate specific tyrosine residues on cytoplasmic receptor domains, thereby creating docking sites for latent, cytoplasmic STAT molecules which bind through their src-homology-2 (SH2) domain. All mammalian STAT proteins bear a conserved signature tyrosine residue near their C-terminus, which becomes phosphorylated by the JAKs. Upon this modification, they dissociate from the receptor complex and immediately dimerise via reciprocal phosphotyrosine (pY)-SH2 domain interactions. With the exception of STAT2, all human STAT proteins form homodimers. In addition, STATs are frequently engaged in heterodimer formation, for example, STAT1:STAT2 and STAT1:STAT3, and the amount of heterodimeric STATs depends on the nature and concentration of the activating ligands.

Due to their large protein size (~180 kDa for the STAT1 dimer), nuclear import of activated STATs requires a carrier-facilitated transport process through the nuclear core complex. Nuclear trafficking of tyrosine-phosphorylated STAT is mediated by importin-α proteins [13]. Tyrosine-phosphorylated STAT1 dimers are translocated as cargo proteins by a mechanism depending on importin α-5:importin-β1 and the small G protein Ran [14–16], whereas nuclear import of STAT3, STAT5 and STAT6 appears to be mediated primarily by interaction with other members of the protein family of karyopherins [17, 18]. Once in the nucleus, the STAT proteins act as classical transcription factors and bind to specific regulatory DNA sequences to activate or repress the transcription of their target genes. All members of the STAT family bind to a palindromic consensus motif termed gamma-interferon activated sequence (GAS) (5′-TTCN$_3$GAA-3′). A notable exception is STAT2, which appears to be defective in DNA binding and instead associates with STAT1 and interferon-regulatory factor 9 (IRF9) in a ternary complex, which is called interferon-stimulated gene factor 3 (ISGF3) [19]. This transcriptionally active complex binds to a distinct direct repeat motif (5′-AGTTTCN$_2$TTTC-3′) termed interferon-α-stimulated response element (ISRE).

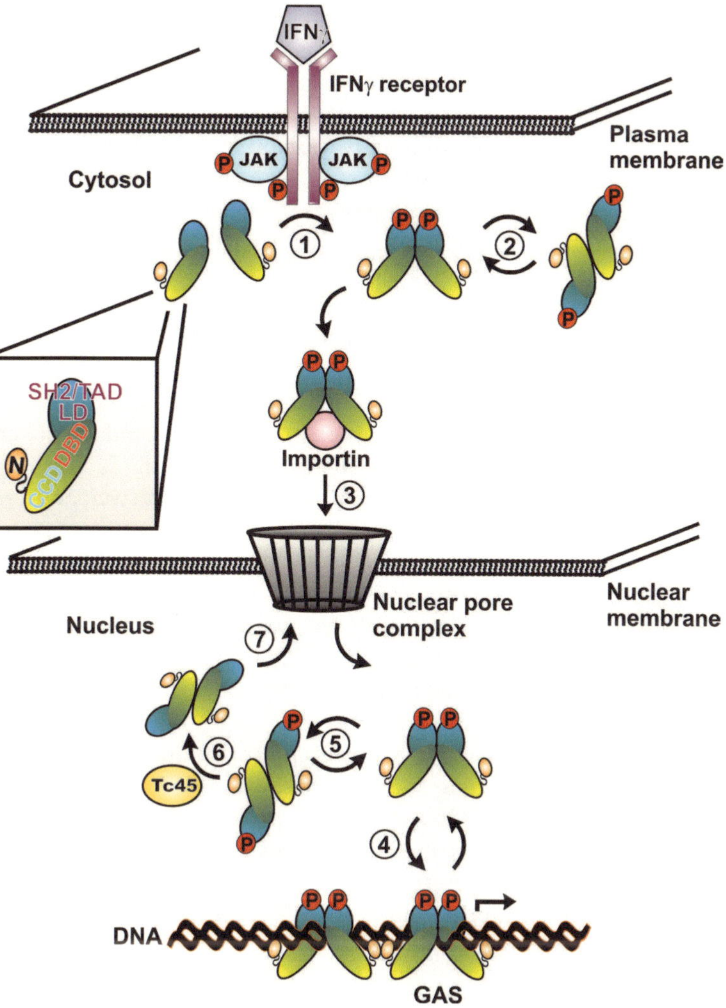

Figure 1.
Model of the interferon-γ-induced JAK/STAT signal pathway depicting the activation-inactivation cycle of STAT1. Binding of IFN-γ to the cell surface receptor triggers JAK-induced tyrosine phosphorylation of STAT1 (1). Through spontaneous dissociation and reassociation, the activated STAT1 molecules constantly oscillate between the parallel and antiparallel dimer conformation (2). Phosphorylated dimers are translocated to the nucleus via binding to importins (3) where they bind to gamma-interferon activated sequence (GAS) motifs, potentially polymerise and induce gene transcription (4). After a conformational shift (5), antiparallel dimers are susceptible to dephosphorylation by the nuclear phosphatase Tc45 (6) and thereafter exit the nucleus (7).

The kinetics of STAT-mediated gene transcription is strictly regulated in both the cytoplasmic and nuclear compartment. The inactivation of nuclear STAT proteins rapidly occurs following nuclear import and initiation of gene transcription. This process has been best studied for the founding member of this family, STAT1. When not contacting DNA, STAT1 dimers undergo a conformational change, which results in the exposure of the critical phosphotyrosine residue at position 701 [20–23]. In this conformation, STAT1 is highly susceptible to dephosphorylation by the nuclear isoform of the T-cell protein tyrosine phosphatase (Tc45) [24–26]. It has been demonstrated that Tc45 induced dephosphorylation is a prerequisite for STAT1 to exit the nucleus [27]. As shown for STAT1 and STAT3, nuclear export is assisted by the exportin CRM1 (chromosome region maintenance 1), which acts in a Ran-dependent manner [28–32]. Back in the cytosol, STATs can then participate in additional cycles of cytoplasmic re-activation, nuclear import and inactivation, depending on the activation status of the cytokine receptor at the plasma membrane [33].

The rapid onset of JAK/STAT signalling is followed by subsequent decay, which includes the inactivation of cytokine receptors and JAKs, leading to a decrease in transcriptional activity. Apart from inactivation by nuclear phosphatases, STAT-mediated signal transduction is tightly controlled by additional negative regulators. A well-studied inhibitory mechanism involves the upregulation of proteins, collectively termed suppressors of cytokine signalling (SOCS) [34, 35]. These inhibitory proteins are components of a classical autoregulatory feedback loop, since most SOCS protein-encoding genes are well-established STAT targets. The SOCS proteins are generally expressed at low levels in resting cells but become rapidly induced after key stimulus exposure. The SOCS protein family comprises SOCS1–7 and the cytokine-inducible SH2-domain-containing protein (CIS), which counteract the JAK/STAT signalling by distinct ways. For example, SOCS1 binds to the catalytic subunit of the receptor-associated JAKs [36], while SOCS3 binds additionally to the receptor [37]. Both processes result in the inhibition of JAK activity and prevent further STAT activation. In contrast, CIS and SOCS2 have been proposed to suppress STAT activation by directly competing with STATs for binding to receptor docking sites [38, 39]. Another antagonistic mechanism involves protein inhibitors of activated STAT (PIAS) [40]. The family members of PIAS proteins are thought to directly bind to activated STAT dimers and show specificity as well as redundancy in their action: PIAS1, PIAS3 and PIASx bind to STAT1, STAT3 and STAT4, respectively [41–43], while PIASy interacts with STAT1 [44]. They employ distinct mechanisms to repress STAT-dependent gene transcription, for example, PIAS1 and PIAS3 block the DNA-binding activity to prevent STATs from binding to their target promoters. In contrast, PIASx and PIASy act as transcriptional co-repressors by recruiting other co-repressors, including histone deacetylases (HDACs) to stop the initiation of transcription. Interestingly, unlike other general negative regulators, PIAS1 does not counteract the entire STAT1-induced gene repertoire but rather selectively inhibits only a subgroup of genes [45].

3. Structure and conformations of dimeric STATs

Mammalian STATs are composed of 750–850 amino acids, and their molecular weights range between 80 and 113 kDa. Biochemical, genetic and structural studies have revealed that STAT family members share the same modular architecture with six conserved functional domains organised in three independently folded structural units (**Figure 2**). The characteristic domains are the amino-terminal domain (ND) involved in protein-protein interactions and the core fragment which is composed of a coiled-coil domain (CCD), DNA-binding domain (DBD), linker domain (LD) and SH2 domain, followed by the carboxy-terminal transactivation domain (TAD) [46, 47]. The N-domain and the transactivation domain are connected to the core fragment through short flexible linkers, of which the C-terminally

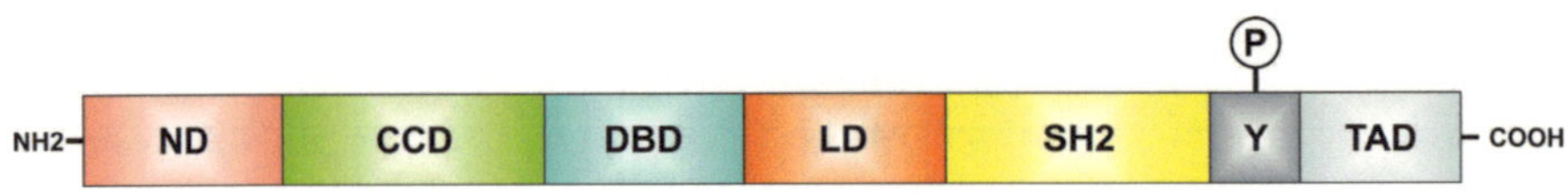

Figure 2.
Domain structure of STATs. STAT proteins are composed of conserved functional domains: ND: amino-terminal domain, CCD: coiled-coil domain, DBD: DNA-binding domain, LD: linker domain, SH2: src-homology-2 domain, TS: phosphotyrosyl tail segment with the specific phosphorylation site, TAD: transactivation domain.

located one harbours the conserved tyrosine residue in a stretch referred to as the phosphotyrosyl tail segment (TS). The overall similar structure and high conservation among the STAT proteins reflect similarities in activation, dimerization and DNA binding. The two most conserved structures are the N-domain and the SH2 domain, both of which facilitate protein interactions, for example, dimerization [48], binding of the transcriptional co-activator CBP/p300 [49] or binding to the receptor. The transactivation domain is intrinsically unstructured and undergoes folding transition upon interaction with transcriptional co-activators [50]. Its residues vary considerably among the STAT family members affording divergent ways to activate individual target genes.

The first crystallographic analyses of STAT proteins revealed the structure of the core fragments of phosphorylated STAT1 and STAT3 lacking the N-domain and parts of the transactivation domain [46, 51] (**Figure 3A–C**). Details of the STAT-DNA interaction showed substantial similarities among the various members of the STAT protein family. The crystal structures of unphosphorylated STAT1 (**Figure 3D–F**) and STAT5A dimers, as well as N-domain dimers of STAT4, greatly extended our general knowledge about the STAT proteins [48, 52, 53]. The original concept of latent STATs existing as cytoplasmic monomers [54] was soon challenged by a growing body of compelling evidence arguing for dimeric conformation prior to stimulus exposure. Crystallographic analyses of STAT1 and STAT5A

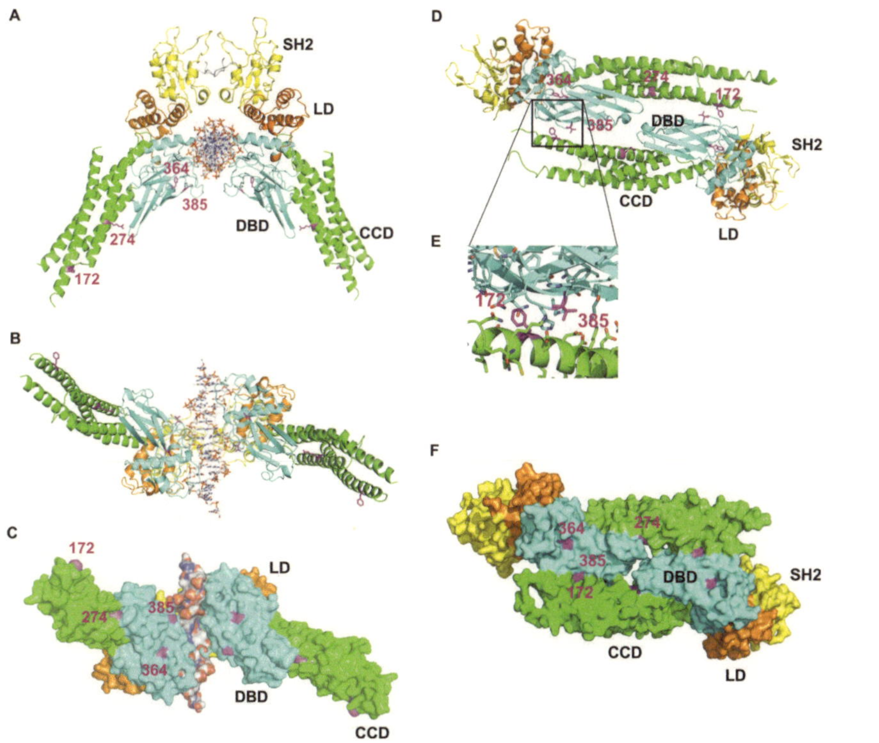

Figure 3.
Localisation of selected gain-of-function mutations within the STAT1 dimer. (A–C): Crystal structure of dimeric STAT1 in parallel conformation bound to DNA including the positions of some important site chains which, when mutated, cause an inborn error. The images show a ribbon diagram (A, B, D, E) or a molecular surface structure (C, F) of a STAT1 core fragment in parallel (A–C) and antiparallel dimer conformation (D–F), respectively. The enlarged section of the ribbon diagram demonstrates the spatial orientation of the residues F172 and T385 (coloured in magenta) in the interdimeric CCD:DBD interface. The selected GOF mutation sites F172, R274, F364 and T385 are marked in magenta. The STAT1 domains are coloured according to the panel in **Figure 2***. CCD: coiled-coil domain. DBD: DNA-binding domain. LD: linker domain. SH2: src-homology-2 domain.*

revealed unphosphorylated protomers self-assembled in a head-to tail alignment where the SH2 domains project from opposite ends of the dimer (**Figure 3D–F**). In this antiparallel conformation, the extended dimeric interface is formed by reciprocal interactions between the coiled-coil domain of one protomer and the DNA-binding domain of its partner protomer (CCD:DBD) [52, 53].

Despite significant efforts, it is still unclear whether a stable dimerization of unphosphorylated monomers is common to all STATs. In addition to unphosphorylated homodimers, experimental data indicate the existence of STAT1:STAT2 and STAT1:STAT3 heterodimers prior to cytokine stimulation [55, 56]. In contrast to the antiparallel alignment in the absence of stimulation, activation of the JAK/STAT signal pathway results in the formation of dimers in parallel conformation, where the tyrosine-phosphorylated protomers arrange themselves in a highly symmetric head-to-head alignment held together by reciprocal phosphotyrosine (pY)-SH2 domain interactions [46, 51] (**Figure 3A–C**). In this conformation, homotypic STAT dimers bind to DNA without the need of further protein-protein interactions between the two protomers. It has been shown that tyrosine-phosphorylated STAT1 must first become dephosphorylated by nuclear phosphatases to be capable of leaving the nucleus to participate in additional rounds of a cytosolic reactivation and nuclear deactivation [27]. In the parallel conformation, the two phosphorylated tyrosine residues are buried in the opposing SH2 domain pockets, thereby protecting STAT1 from being dephosphorylated. By the conformational rearrangement of the STAT1 dimer from a parallel to an antiparallel alignment, the critical phosphotyrosine residues are subjected to enzymatic dephosphorylation [23].

The molecular details of the transition between the parallel and antiparallel STAT1 dimer conformation are still controversial. Initially, a model was proposed in which the N-terminal domains dimerise and keep the dimer partners held together, while the monomer's core domains rotate around each other after phosphotyrosine-SH2 disjunction [22]. The alternative mechanism, widely accepted today, describes the conformational reorientation as achieved by spontaneous dissociation of the tyrosine-phosphorylated dimer into isolated monomers and their reassociation in antiparallel alignment [20, 57]. Studies indicate that STAT1 constantly oscillates between the two dimer conformations, and the abundance of each conformer is determined by the level of tyrosine phosphorylation. While unphosphorylated molecules exist in monomeric or dimeric, antiparallel conformation, there is a conformational equilibrium between phosphorylated dimers in parallel and antiparallel alignment [20].

4. Nucleocytoplasmic shuttling and transcriptional activity

Initially, STAT proteins were considered to function as latent transcription factors, which translocate to the nucleus and induce gene transcription exclusively in response to stimulus exposure. However, STAT1 and STAT3 were found to be present in the nucleus independent of tyrosine phosphorylation [33, 58, 59]. It became evident that, in contrast to phosphorylated STATs that are actively transported into the nucleus, the nuclear import of unphosphorylated STATs is facilitated by direct interactions with protein components constituting the nuclear pore complex [28]. This carrier-free translocation follows the concentration gradient across the nuclear envelope and, as facilitated diffusion, does not depend on metabolic energy. Thus, STAT proteins are constantly shuttling between the cytoplasmic and nuclear compartment, irrespective of their activation status. For some STAT family members, for example, STAT1, STAT2, STAT3 and STAT6, it has been shown that they play important roles in facilitating gene expression in the absence of stimuli and tyrosine phosphorylation [60–64]. In principle, unphosphorylated STAT1 is able to bind to

DNA, but its binding activity is 200-fold lower than that of activated STAT1 and, therefore, may not have any physiological relevance as a DNA-binding protein without the recruitment of cofactors [20]. In line, unphosphorylated STAT1 was found in a complex with interferon-regulatory factor 1 (IRF1) to bind DNA at the promoter of the *low molecular mass polypeptide 2* (*LMP2*) gene, which contains overlapping binding sites for both transcription factors [65]. The *LMP2* gene encodes a component of the 20S proteasome and is induced by stimulation of cells with IFN-γ, but it is also expressed at low levels in the absence of cytokines [66]. From these experiments, it became clear that unphosphorylated STAT1 functions as a transcription factor, since it is directly responsible for constitutive *LMP2* expression, but it is rapidly replaced by activated STAT1 dimers in response to IFN-γ stimulation [65].

More recently, it was reported that, in comparison to STAT1-deficient knockout animals, the pathogene *Listeria monocytogenes* grows less robustly in knockin mice expressing the $Y^{701}F$ mutant, which is unable to be tyrosine phosphorylated, indicating a potential contribution of unphosphorylated STAT1 to innate antibacterial immunity [67]. Due to a positive autoregulatory loop of STAT1 signalling, expression of unphosphorylated STAT1 molecules is greatly increased after activation of STAT1. While the phosphorylation in response to IFNs lasts only for several hours, newly synthesised unphosphorylated STAT1 persists for several days and results in enhanced signal transduction when the cells are thereafter re-exposed to low doses of IFN [68].

5. Serine phosphorylation and its effect on transcriptional activity

Apart from canonical, tyrosine phosphorylation STAT-driven transcription is also regulated by a number of posttranslational modifications, including serine phosphorylation and sumoylation. All STATs except STAT2 can become phosphorylated at least at one serine residue embedded in a proline-rich sequence in the C-terminal transactivation domain [69]. An evolutionary conserved phosphorylation site includes Ser 727 in STAT1 and STAT3, Ser 721 in STAT4, Ser 725 in STAT5A, Ser 730 in STAT5B and Ser 756 in STAT6 [70, 71]. The maximal transcriptional activity and biological effects of at least STAT1, STAT3, and STAT4, and possibly also STAT5A, require both tyrosine and serine phosphorylation [70, 72–75]. This was corroborated by infection experiments with mice unable to become phosphorylated at STAT1 Ser 727. Mice expressing STAT1 $S^{727}A$ died when challenged with high doses of the intracellular pathogen *Listeria monocytogenes*, whereas 80% of the wild-type littermates survived [72]. In the case of STAT1, a variety of signals cause the phosphorylation of Ser 727 and multiple candidate serine/threonine kinases have been implicated in this process. For example, interferons induce serine phosphorylation in addition to prior tyrosine phosphorylation. It was reported that, for canonical serine phosphorylation, STAT1 needs to be assembled into chromatin-bound transcriptional complexes and that the responsible kinase itself is similarly associated with DNA [76]. In this light, it was proposed that STAT1 recruits the cyclin-dependent kinase 8 (CDK8) to IFN-γ-driven target genes, which provides the kinase activity [77].

The need for serine phosphorylation to enhance transcriptional activity of STAT1 varies with different target genes and cell types, suggesting a complexity, which is not yet fully understood [72, 78]. It is hypothesised that STAT1 serine phosphorylation provides an extra supply of IFN-γ-induced gene products that are critical for full protection against pathogens [72]. Signals such as bacterial lipopolysaccharide (LPS) or mediators of inflammation and cellular stress exclusively stimulate the phosphorylation of serine 727, independent of tyrosine phosphorylation [79]. This modification takes place in the cytosol and involves the p38 mitogen-activated protein kinase (MAPK) pathway [80, 81]. It has been proposed that the biological relevance of serine phosphorylation is to prime STAT1 for an increased transcriptional response once IFN-γ provides the stimulus for tyrosine phosphorylation [78], as observed for macrophage activation.

An important paper from the Vinkemeier lab demonstrated that the activity of STAT1 is inhibited by conjugation to small ubiquitin-like modifier (SUMO), which is added to Lys 703 [82]. Although only a small fraction of the intracellular, unphosphorylated STAT1 pool is sumoylated, the modification by SUMO interferes with the formation of paracrystalline arrays in the nucleus, which sequester activated STAT1 molecules. SUMO conjugation diminishes the activity of STAT1 by interference with tyrosine phosphorylation and, in addition, solubilizes the highly dynamic paracrystals in cytokine-stimulated cells [83].

6. Mechanisms of STAT1 DNA binding

Sequence-specific DNA binding of STAT proteins is a prerequisite for their function as cytokine-driven transcriptional regulators. STATs interact with high-affinity binding sites on DNA through their DNA-binding domain, which shows the general architecture of an immunoglobulin fold [46, 47]. The crystal structure of DNA-bound STAT1 revealed that the transcription factor engages in several interactions with the phosphodiester backbone of the DNA, but makes relatively few base-specific contacts, for example, through the residues Asp 460 and Lys 336 in the major and through Glu 421 in the minor groove [46]. Each STAT protomer binds to a half-site of a palindromic consensus motif termed gamma-interferon activated sequence (GAS). STAT1, STAT3, STAT4 and STAT5 bind to half-sites spacing two or three base pairs (5′-TTCN$_{2-3}$GAA-′3), while STAT6 favours a four nucleotide spacer within the palindrome [84, 85]. The nucleotides between and around the core palindrome impart some level of specificity.

The implication of impaired DNA-binding activity became evident, when STAT1 mutants were engineered by substituting numerous residues within the DNA-binding domain that potentially make contacts with the phosphodiester backbone of the DNA. The introduction of positive, negative or neutral charges was intended to increase or reduce electrostatic interactions between STAT1 and DNA, respectively. A STAT1 mutant termed STAT1 DNA^{minus}, in which negative charges were introduced by substituting aspartic acid (Asp) for valine (Val) at position 426 (Val^{426}Asp) and threonine at position 427 (Thr^{427}Asp), was normally tyrosine phosphorylated in response to IFN-γ but essentially lost its DNA-binding activity [27]. The STAT1 DNA^{minus} mutant was highly susceptible to inactivation by the nuclear phosphatase Tc45 and failed to accumulate in the nucleus. In contrast, the mutant STAT1 DNA^{plus} (Thr^{327}Arg; Val^{426}His; Thr^{427}His) was capable of strongly binding to both specific GAS sites and nonspecific DNA sequences with nearly equal affinity. This mutant lost its discrimination for GAS sites and, due to its hindered dissociation from DNA, resisted dephosphorylation, resulting in prolonged nuclear accumulation [27]. These and additional experiments indicated that DNA binding determines the accumulation of STAT1 in the nucleus. This assumption was corroborated by the finding that high-affinity DNA binding reduces the dissociation rate of STAT1 dimers from DNA and impairs the interdimeric exchange of their protomers in the presence of DNA [57].

In contrast to STAT1 DNA^{plus}, substitution of two glutamic acid residues (Glu^{411}Ala; Glu^{421}Lys) generates a double mutant, which maintains the discrimination between GAS and nonspecific sites. However, STAT1-DNA complexes are stabilised independent of the nucleotide sequence, leading to persistent and enhanced tyrosine phosphorylation and prolonged nuclear accumulation [86]. The presence of negatively charged residues at these positions is critical for the release of STAT1 from DNA. IFN-γ-induced expression of reporter genes and endogenous target genes is dramatically reduced in cells expressing STAT1 DNA^{plus}, STAT1 Glu^{411}Ala or STAT1 Glu^{421}Lys [27, 86]. In summary, these data revealed the significance of sequence-specific DNA binding and fast dissociation from DNA for efficient STAT1-mediated gene regulation. An impaired dissociation of STAT1 from genomic DNA not only interferes with the continuous search for GAS sites but also prevents fast nucleocytoplasmic shuttling and full transcriptional activity of STAT1.

Early studies on the DNA binding of STATs revealed that their binding sites can extend over two or more adjacent consensus motifs and that activated STAT1, STAT3, STAT4 and STAT5 dimers can interact in homotypic fashion to polymerise on such DNA sequences, that is form tetramers or even higher order oligomers [48, 87–91]. GAS motifs linked in tandem orientation have been identified in various STAT-driven target genes, including, for example, those encoding IFN-γ [90], interleukin 2 receptor α (IL-2Rα) [87, 88], perforin [92], cytokine-inducible SH2-containing protein (CIS) [93], α2-macroglobulin (α2-M) [91], and glycosylation-dependent cell adhesion molecule 1 (GlyCam1) [94]. The synergistic recognition of DNA, generally referred to as cooperative DNA binding, is mediated by the conserved N-terminal domain of the STAT proteins. It was shown that deletion or mutation of the STAT N-terminus abolishes cooperative dimer-dimer interactions [48, 89–91, 95].

Analysis of the crystal structure of the N-domain dimer has indicated an extensive interface involving interactions between hydrophobic residues [96]. Targeted mutagenesis has revealed an orthologue residue (Phe 77 in STAT1 and Phe 81 in STAT5A/B, respectively) as physiologically most relevant for the oligomerisation of STAT proteins [95, 96]. Substitution of alanine for the critical phenylalanine in STAT1 does not overtly affect DNA binding on a single GAS site in response to IFN-γ but severely impairs tetramerisation [95, 97]. The cooperative binding of STAT1 dimers strongly increases their DNA-binding affinity [89]. Such interactions do not require high-affinity GAS sites linked in tandem orientation. *In vitro* studies have revealed the recruitment of multiple STAT1 dimers to a single GAS site adjacent to low-affinity or even GAS-unrelated sequences [95]. Thus, N-domain interactions of DNA-bound STAT1 molecules greatly expand the repertoire of potential STAT1-regulated IFN-γ target genes. An *in silico* analysis revealed that although single GAS sites frequently occur in the mouse genome, GAS sites linked in tandem orientation are rare and may not be enriched in IFN-γ target genes [97]. Paradoxically, a genome-wide transcriptional analysis revealed that STAT1-mediated cooperative DNA binding is indispensable for IFN-γ signalling, since the IFN-γ response is essentially lost in murine cells expressing the STAT1 F^{77}A mutant [97]. Furthermore, cooperativity-deficient STAT1 F^{77}A showed a pervasive promoter recruitment defect at GAS-containing IFN-γ-driven but not IFN-α/β-driven genes. It has, therefore, been proposed that STAT1 tetramerisation or polymerisation originates from a GAS site and then proceeds with loose additional requirements for adjacent sequences [97]. Infection experiments have highlighted the physiological relevance of STAT1 tetramerisation. *Listeria monocytogenes* infection of STAT1 F^{77}A-expressing mice revealed a severe defect in antibacterial immunity. The STAT1 cooperativity-deficient animals succumbed more easily than their wild-type littermates [97].

The crystal structure of the unphosphorylated STAT1 dimer indicates that the dimerisation interface is composed of the phenylalanine residue 172 in the coiled-coil domain of one protomer, which reciprocally is inserted into a pocket in the DNA-binding domain of its partner molecule. This pocket is created by the residues Q340, L383, G384, T385, H406, L407 and Q408 [52]. Several GOF mutations have been identified at this interdimeric interface [98, 99]. Studies on the molecular basis of these point mutations underscore the paramount importance of the conformational shift for STAT1-driven gene expression [98]. The critical phenylalanine residue 172 is in close proximity (7 Å) to the threonine residue 385 at the surface of the partner protomer (**Figure 3E**). Its substitution impedes the reciprocal interactions between the coiled-coil and DNA-binding domain of the two interacting STAT1 molecules, thereby negatively affecting the stability of the antiparallel dimer conformation. Shifting the conformational equilibrium towards the parallel conformation buries the critical tyrosine residue 701 inside the SH2 domain and, thus, prevents access for nuclear phosphatases.

Another interesting phenotype was reported from the targeted mutagenesis of the phenylalanine residue 364. The crystal structure indicates that this residue locates in the centre of the DNA-binding domain and contributes to the gross structural alignment of this domain (**Figure 3**). The $F^{364}A$ mutant is characterised by tyrosine hyper-phosphorylation in response to stimulation of cells with IFN-γ, most likely because of its hampered interaction with the Tc45 phosphatase and, in addition, a significantly reduced DNA-binding activity. The data suggest that Phe 364 is crucial for stabilising the antiparallel dimer and, in addition, for recognising DNA-binding sites. When assessed for its ability to induce endogenous STAT1-regulated genes, the mutant unexpectedly shows a well-preserved transcriptional activity. Remarkably, it appears that a shift in the equilibrium towards the parallel dimer conformation can compensate for a critical impairment in high-affinity DNA binding, restoring nearly full transcriptional activity at IFN-γ-induced target genes [21].

7. Phenotypes of patients with inborn errors of human STAT1

Regulation of the JAK-STAT signalling pathway is most critical, and dysfunctions in this pathway are associated with various immune disorders and cancer. Either the loss of STAT transcriptional activity or uncontrolled constitutive, prolonged activity can have devastating effects. Recent progress in the genetic dissection of various human infectious diseases has shed light on the inborn errors of human STAT1-mediated immunity. In the latest version of the publicly accessible section of the Human Gene Mutation Database (HGMD), more than 40 missense/nonsense mutations in the *Stat1* gene have been listed as disease-causing mutations. These include mutations with (i) autosomal recessive (AR) complete STAT1 deficiency, (ii) AR partial STAT1 deficiency, (iii) autosomal dominant (AD) STAT1 deficiency and (iv) AD gain-of-function activity. Biallelic and even monoallelic loss-of-function (LOF) mutations have been associated with lethal or milder pathogenesis of intramacrophagic bacterial and viral diseases. In addition, STAT1 LOF mutations have been identified in the rare syndrome of Mendelian susceptibility to mycobacterial disease (MSMD), which is characterised by infections with weakly virulent mycobacteria in otherwise healthy individuals. Patients with immunological defects caused by gain-of-function (GOF) mutations suffer from autoimmunity and recurrent or persistent infections of nails, skin and mucous membranes with the opportunistic yeast pathogen *Candida albicans*, referred to as chronic mucocutaneous candidiasis (CMC) [100–102] (**Table 1**).

Studying the structural and functional impact of STAT1 missense mutations has greatly contributed to our current understanding of cytokine-regulated transcriptional activity. To decipher the underlying molecular mechanisms of the known STAT1-mediated immunodeficiencies, the pathogenic amino-acid substitutions need to be assigned to the structural changes they induce in the context of intra- and intermolecular interactions [112]. When mapped to the crystal structure, it becomes evident that the occurrence of disease-causing mutations is unevenly distributed among the different STAT1 domains. It appears that the preferential

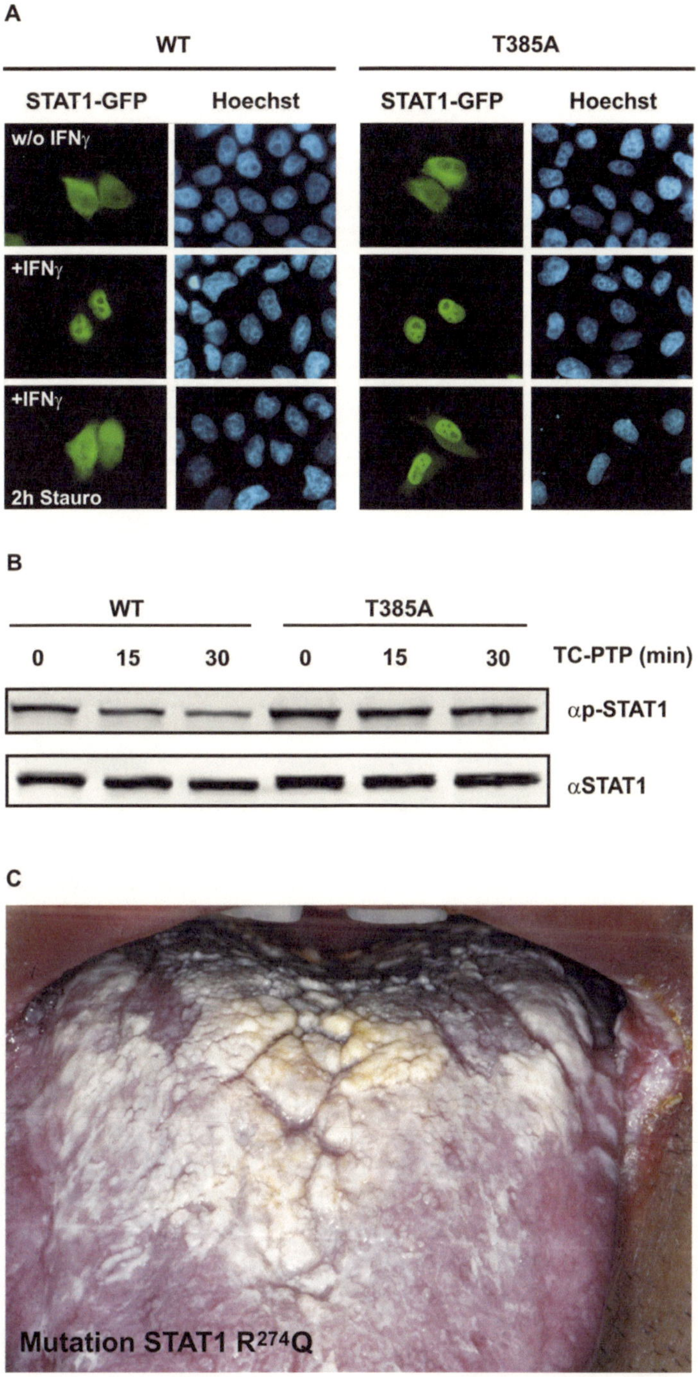

Figure 4.
Phenotype of clinically relevant STAT1 GOF mutations. (A, B): Characterisation of the STAT1 mutation T^{385}A. (A) Localisation of fusion proteins of green-fluorescent protein-tagged STAT1 in reconstituted U3A cells expressing recombinant wild-type STAT1 or STAT1 T^{385}A. Exposure to the kinase inhibitor staurosporine resulted in the loss of IFN-γ-induced nuclear accumulation of wild-type STAT1, whereas, in contrast, the STAT1 point mutant showed a significantly prolonged nuclear residence. (B) Impaired tyrosine dephosphorylation of the GOF mutant, as shown by Western blotting. Incubation of protein extracts from STAT1-reconstituted U3A cells with the STAT1-specific nuclear phosphatase TC-PTP (Tc45) led to rapid dephosphorylation of wild-type STAT1, while the level of tyrosine phosphorylation was prolonged in the T^{385}A mutant. (C) Intraoral chronic mucocutaneous candidiasis in a patient carrying the heterozygous STAT1 GOF mutation R^{274}Q.

	Domain/ region affected	Main cellular phenotype	Predominant clinical phenotype	References (incomplete)
AR complete STAT1 deficiency	ND, SH2	No STAT1-dependent response to IFN-α/β, IFN-γ, IFN-λ, IL-27	Life-threatening intracellular bacterial (mostly mycobacteria) and viral (mostly herpes) diseases	[103–105]
AR partial STAT1 deficiency	ND, CCD, TS	Impaired STAT1-dependent response to IFN-α/β, IFN-γ, IFN-λ, IL-27	Mild intracellular bacterial (mostly mycobacteria) and viral (mostly herpes) diseases	[106, 107]
AD LOF STAT1 disorder	CCD, DBD, SH2, TS	Impaired STAT1-dependent response to IFN-γ, IL-27	Mendelian susceptibility to mycobacterial disease (MSMD)	[108, 109, 116]
AD GOF STAT1 disorder	CCD, DBD	Enhanced STAT1-dependent response to IFN-α/β, IFN-γ, IFN-λ, IL-27, IL-6, IL-21, impaired IL-17-mediated T-cell immunity	Chronic mucocutaneous candidiasis (CMC) Autoimmunity	[99, 110, 111]

AD, autosomal dominant; AR, autosomal recessive; CCD, coiled-coil domain; DBD, DNA-binding domain; GOF, gain-of-function; LOF, loss-of-function; ND, amino-terminal domain; SH2, src-homology-2 domain; TS, tail segment.

Table 1.
Inborn errors of human STAT1-mediated immunity.

localisation of LOF mutations is less well defined as compared to the more restricted localisation of GOF mutations. The critical LOF substitutions are widely scattered in the coiled-coil, DNA-binding and SH2 domains, as well as in the tail segment. In contrast, the GOF mutations identified so far are exclusively clustered in the coiled-coil and DNA-binding domains. The crystal structure of tyrosine-phosphorylated, DNA-bound STAT1 shows that the coiled-coil domain prominently protrudes outward [46]. Therefore, it was initially postulated that the coiled-coil domain may function as a docking site for transcription factors and coactivators to cooperatively facilitate STAT1-dependent gene transcription and that the GOF mutations in this domain may enhance these interactions. Typically, pathogenic GOF mutations cluster in structural areas of the STAT1 protein, which markedly affect the regulation of its transcriptional activity. As described above, the conformational rearrangement from the parallel to the antiparallel dimer conformation is a prerequisite for the inactivation of STAT1 and requires, as a *conditio sine qua non,* the dissociation into monomers. Monomeric STAT1 spontaneously reassociates into either the parallel or antiparallel conformation. In the parallel alignment, STAT1 regains its DNA-binding activity with the chance of participating in another round of transcriptional initiation of target genes. It appears that the antiparallel conformation of the STAT1 dimer is the substrate for the highly active Tc45 phosphatase, which rapidly dephosphorylates the critical tyrosine residue 701 followed by nuclear export of the now transcriptionally inactive molecule. As described above, the formation of the antiparallel dimer is facilitated by reciprocal interactions between the coiled-coil and the DNA-binding domain and, thus, it is not surprising that mutations in this critical area affect the stability of this complex.

Experimental data revealed that the two point mutants STAT1 $F^{172}W$ and $T^{385}A$ are resistant against dephosphorylation by the Tc45 phosphatase, which results in prolonged nuclear accumulation in cells exposed to IFN-γ (**Figure 4A**, **B**) [113]. The resulting phenotype is associated with enhanced tyrosine phosphorylation in response to various cytokine stimuli, including IFN-α, IFN-γ, IL-6, IL-21 and IL-27 [23, 110, 113–115]. The functional characterisation of the disease-causing interface mutations has demonstrated sequence-specific requirements for differential gene expression of endogenous IFN-γ target genes. The expression of genes with a classical GAS consensus-binding motif, including *interferon-regulatory factor 1* (*irf1*), *guanylate-binding protein 1* (*gbp1*) and *monokine induced by interferon gamma 1* (*mig1*), is virtually unaffected by these mutations. In contrast, transcription of genes, such as *CXC motif chemokine 10* (*cxcl10*) and *monocyte chemotactic protein 1* (*mcp1/cxcl9*) is greatly increased, which have a "one-and-a-half-GAS" element in their promoters, that is, half of the palindromic motif adjacent to the GAS site [113]. The superiority of the STAT1 mutants as transcriptional activators appears to directly reflect their enhanced binding as tetramers to these "one-and-a-half-GAS" sequences. The increased DNA binding for these mutants contributes to their pathologically elevated level of tyrosine phosphorylation. However, numerous disease-associated GOF mutations are not directly located at the surface of the interdimeric interface but rather disturb the gross architecture of this interface (**Figure 3**).

A prominent and well-studied example is the GOF mutation resulting from the exchange of the arginine 274 residue in the coiled-coil domain (**Figure 4C**). A change in the local structure induced by this substitution may impair the stability of the antiparallel dimer. Consistently, a genome-wide expression profile indicated that the pathogenic $R^{274}Q$ mutation increased the IFN-γ-induced transcriptional activity of STAT1 but overall retained its sequence specificity [98]. In other words, the mutation increases the expression rate of STAT1 target genes but does not dramatically change its repertoire. However, the molecular mechanisms of this GOF mutation are not fully understood. In particular, it is unclear whether this missense mutation affects the kinetics of JAK-induced phosphorylation or, alternatively, its dephosphorylation rate.

8. Concluding remarks

Activation at the IFN receptor and sequence-specific, cooperative DNA binding are key features of STAT1 signal transduction. Cytoplasmic and nuclear activities are functionally coupled by repetitive cycles of STAT1 phosphorylation and dephosphorylation. This highly dynamic activation-inactivation circuit is controlled by a shift between the parallel and antiparallel dimer conformers. Missense mutations in either the coiled-coil or DNA-binding domain destabilising the antiparallel dimer critically interfere with the equilibrium between the two conformers. Genetic variations affecting this intradimeric interface result in enhanced cytokine-induced gene expression and cause severe immunodeficiencies in heterozygous mutation carriers.

Acknowledgements

We apologise to many researchers in the field whose primary publications and important contributions could not be cited, due to space restrains. We thank Professor Timo Buhl, University of Göttingen, for providing the photograph of the patient with the heterozygous STAT1 GOF mutation. The authors gratefully acknowledge the excellent technical assistance of Anke Gregus and Heike Hühn. This work was supported by funds from the Deutsche Forschungsgemeinschaft and the Nachlass Frau Lore Grun from the University Medical Centre of Göttingen.

Author details

Roswitha Nast, Julia Staab and Thomas Meyer*
Department of Psychosomatic Medicine and Psychotherapy, University of Göttingen, Göttingen, Germany

*Address all correspondence to: thomas.meyer@med.uni-goettingen.de

References

[1] Darnell JE, Kerr IM, Stark GR. JAK-STAT pathways and transcriptional activation in response to IFNs and other extracellular signaling proteins. Science. 1994;**264**:1415-1421

[2] Wang Y, Levy DE. Comparative evolutionary genomics of the STAT family of transcription factors. JAK-STAT Journal. 2012;**1**:23-33

[3] de Mendoza A, Sebé-Pedrós A, Šestak MS, Matejcic M, Torruella G, Domazet-Loso T, et al. Transcription factor evolution in eukaryotes and the assembly of the regulatory toolkit in multicellular lineages. Proceedings of the National Academy of Sciences of the United States of America. 2013;**110**:E4858-E4866

[4] Wang Y, Levy DE. *C. elegans* STAT cooperates with DAF-7/TGF-beta signaling to repress dauer formation. Current Biology. 2006;**16**:89-94

[5] Yan R, Small S, Desplan C, Dearolf CR, Darnell JE. Identification of a *stat* gene that functions in Drosophila development. Cell. 1996;**84**:421-430

[6] Barillas-Mury C, Han YS, Seeley D, Kafatos FC. *Anopheles gambiae* Ag-STAT, a new insect member of the STAT family, is activated in response to bacterial infection. The EMBO Journal. 1999;**18**:959-967

[7] Pascal A, Riou JF, Carron C, Boucaut JC, Umbhauer M. Cloning and developmental expression of STAT5 in *Xenopus laevis*. Mechanisms of Development. 2001;**106**:171-174

[8] Oates AC, Wollberg P, Pratt SJ, Paw BH, Johnson SL, Ho RK, et al. Zebrafish STAT3 is expressed in restricted tissues during embryogenesis and STAT1 rescues cytokine signaling in a STAT1-deficient human cell line. Developmental Dynamics. 1999;**215**:352-370

[9] Lewis RS, Ward AC. Conservation, duplication and divergence of the zebrafish *stat5* genes. Gene. 2004;**338**:65-74

[10] Abroun S, Saki N, Ahmadvand M, Asghari F, Salari F, Rahim F. STATs: An old story, yet mesmerizing. Cell Journal. 2015;**17**:395-411

[11] Levy DE, Darnell JE. STATs: Transcriptional control and biological impact. Nature Reviews. Molecular Cell Biology. 2002;**3**:651-662

[12] Hu X, Ivashkiv LB. Cross-regulation of signaling pathways by interferon-gamma: Implications for immune responses and autoimmune diseases. Immunity. 2009;**31**:539-550

[13] Meyer T, Vinkemeier U. STAT nuclear translocation: Potential for pharmacological intervention. Expert Opinion on Therapeutic Targets. 2007;**11**:1355-1365

[14] Fagerlund R, Mélen K, Kinnunen L, Julkunen I. Arginine/lysine-rich nuclear localization signals mediate interactions between dimeric STATs and importin alpha5. The Journal of Biological Chemistry. 2002;**277**:30072-30078

[15] Sekimoto T, Imamoto N, Nakajima K, Hirano T, Yoneda Y. Extracellular signal-dependent nuclear import of STAT1 is mediated by nuclear pore-targeting complex formation with NPI-1, but not Rch1. The EMBO Journal. 1997;**16**:7067-7077

[16] Sekimoto T, Nakajima K, Tachibana T, Hirano T, Yoneda Y. Interferon-gamma-dependent nuclear import of STAT1 is mediated by the GTPase activity of Ran/TC4. The Journal of Biological Chemistry. 1996;**271**:31017-31020

[17] Ma J, Cao X. Regulation of STAT3 nuclear import by importin alpha5

and importin alpha7 via two different functional sequence elements. Cellular Signalling. 2006;**18**:1117-1126

[18] Ushijima R, Sakaguchi N, Kano A, Maruyama A, Miyamoto Y, Sekimoto T, et al. Extracellular signal-dependent nuclear import of STAT3 is mediated by various importin alphas. Biochemical and Biophysical Research Communications. 2005;**330**:880-886

[19] Bluyssen HA, Levy DE. STAT2 is a transcriptional activator that requires sequence-specific contacts provided by STAT1 and p48 for stable interaction with DNA. The Journal of Biological Chemistry. 1997;**272**:4600-4605

[20] Wenta N, Strauss H, Meyer S, Vinkemeier U. Tyrosine phosphorylation regulates the partitioning of STAT1 between different dimer conformations. Proceedings of the National Academy of Sciences of the United States of America. 2008;**105**:9238-9243

[21] Staab J, Herrmann-Lingen C, Meyer T. A rapid conformational rearrangement of STAT1 dimers is required for termination rather than for amplification of interferon-γ signaling. JAK-STAT Journal. 2013;**2**:e23576

[22] Mertens C, Zhong M, Krishnaraj R, Zou W, Chen X, Darnell JE. Dephosphorylation of phosphotyrosine on STAT1 dimers requires extensive spatial reorientation of the monomers facilitated by the N-terminal domain. Genes & Development. 2006;**20**:3372-3381

[23] Zhong M, Henriksen MA, Takeuchi K, Schaefer O, Liu B, ten Hoeve J, et al. Implications of an antiparallel dimeric structure of nonphosphorylated STAT1 for the activation-inactivation cycle. Proceedings of the National Academy of Sciences of the United States of America. 2005;**102**:3966-3971

[24] ten Hoeve J, de Jesus Ibarra-Sanchez M, Fu Y, Zhu W, Tremblay M, David M, et al. Identification of a nuclear STAT1 protein tyrosine phosphatase. Molecular and Cellular Biology. 2002;**22**:5662-5668

[25] Yamamoto T, Sekine Y, Kashima K, Kubota A, Sato N, Aoki N, et al. The nuclear isoform of protein-tyrosine phosphatase TC-PTP regulates interleukin-6-mediated signaling pathway through STAT3 dephosphorylation. Biochemical and Biophysical Research Communications. 2002;**297**:811-817

[26] Pelzel C, Begitt A, Wenta N, Vinkemeier U. Evidence against a role for β-arrestin1 in STAT1 dephosphorylation and the inhibition of interferon-γ signaling. Molecular Cell. 2013;**50**:149-156

[27] Meyer T, Marg A, Lemke P, Wiesner B, Vinkemeier U. DNA binding controls inactivation and nuclear accumulation of the transcription factor Stat1. Genes & Development. 2003;**17**:1992-2005

[28] Marg A, Shan Y, Meyer T, Meissner T, Brandenburg M, Vinkemeier U. Nucleocytoplasmic shuttling by nucleoporins Nup153 and Nup214 and CRM1-dependent nuclear export control the subcellular distribution of latent STAT1. The Journal of Cell Biology. 2004;**165**:823-833

[29] Bhattacharya S, Schindler C. Regulation of STAT3 nuclear export. The Journal of Clinical Investigation. 2003;**111**:553-559

[30] Sato N, Tsuruma R, Imoto S, Sekine Y, Muromoto R, Sugiyama K, et al. Nuclear retention of STAT3 through the coiled-coil domain regulates its activity. Biochemical and Biophysical Research Communications. 2005;**336**:617-624

[31] Lödige I, Marg A, Wiesner B, Malecová B, Oelgeschläger T, Vinkemeier U. Nuclear export determines the cytokine sensitivity of STAT transcription factors. The Journal of Biological Chemistry. 2005;**280**:43087-43099

[32] Rodriguez JJ, Parisien JP, Horvath CM. Nipah virus V protein evades alpha and gamma interferons by preventing STAT1 and STAT2 activation and nuclear accumulation. Journal of Virology. 2002;**76**:11476-11483

[33] Meyer T, Begitt A, Lödige I, van Rossum M, Vinkemeier U. Constitutive and IFN-gamma-induced nuclear import of STAT1 proceed through independent pathways. The EMBO Journal. 2002;**21**:344-354

[34] Linossi EM, Babon JJ, Hilton DJ, Nicholson SE. Suppression of cytokine signaling: The SOCS perspective. Cytokine & Growth Factor Reviews. 2013;**24**:241-248

[35] Linossi EM, Nicholson SE. Kinase inhibition, competitive binding and proteasomal degradation: Resolving the molecular function of the suppressor of cytokine signaling (SOCS) proteins. Immunological Reviews. 2015;**266**:123-133

[36] Endo TA, Masuhara M, Yokouchi M, Suzuki R, Sakamoto H, Mitsui K, et al. A new protein containing an SH2 domain that inhibits JAK kinases. Nature. 1997;**387**:921-924

[37] Kershaw NJ, Murphy JM, Liau NP, Varghese LN, Laktyushin A, Whitlock EL, et al. SOCS3 binds specific receptor-JAK complexes to control cytokine signaling by direct kinase inhibition. Nature Structural & Molecular Biology. 2013;**20**:469-476

[38] Verdier F, Chrétien S, Muller O, Varlet P, Yoshimura A, Gisselbrecht S, et al. Proteasomes regulate erythropoietin receptor and signal transducer and activator of transcription 5 (STAT5) activation. Possible involvement of the ubiquitinated CIS protein. The Journal of Biological Chemistry. 1998;**273**:28185-28190

[39] Matsumoto A, Masuhara M, Mitsui K, Yokouchi M, Ohtsubo M, Misawa H, et al. CIS, a cytokine inducible SH2 protein, is a target of the JAK-STAT5 pathway and modulates STAT5 activation. Blood. 1997;**89**:3148-3154

[40] Shuai K. Regulation of cytokine signaling pathways by PIAS proteins. Cell Research. 2006;**16**:196-202

[41] Liu B, Liao J, Rao X, Kushner SA, Chung CD, Chang DD, et al. Inhibition of STAT1-mediated gene activation by PIAS1. Proceedings of the National Academy of Sciences of the United States of America. 1998;**95**:10626-10631

[42] Chung CD, Liao J, Liu B, Rao X, Jay P, Berta P, et al. Specific inhibition of STAT3 signal transduction by PIAS3. Science. 1997;**278**:1803-1805

[43] Arora T, Liu B, He H, Kim J, Murphy TL, Murphy KM, et al. PIASx is a transcriptional co-repressor of signal transducer and activator of transcription 4. The Journal of Biological Chemistry. 2003;**278**:21327-21330

[44] Liu B, Gross M, ten Hoeve J, Shuai K. A transcriptional corepressor of STAT1 with an essential LXXLL signature motif. Proceedings of the National Academy of Sciences of the United States of America. 2001;**98**:3203-3207

[45] Liu B, Mink S, Wong KA, Stein N, Getman C, Dempsey PW, et al. PIAS1 selectively inhibits interferon-inducible genes and is important in innate immunity. Nature Immunology. 2004;**5**:891-898

[46] Chen X, Vinkemeier U, Zhao Y, Jeruzalmi D, Darnell JE, Kuriyan J. Crystal structure of a tyrosine phosphorylated STAT1 dimer bound to DNA. Cell. 1998;**93**:827-839

[47] Horvath CM, Wen Z, Darnell JE. A STAT protein domain that determines DNA sequence recognition suggests a novel DNA-binding domain. Genes & Development. 1995;**9**:984-994

[48] Vinkemeier U, Moarefi I, Darnell JE, Kuriyan J. Structure of the amino-terminal protein interaction domain of STAT4. Science. 1998;**279**:1048-1052

[49] Zhang JJ, Vinkemeier U, Gu W, Chakravarti D, Horvath CM, Darnell JE. Two contact regions between STAT1 and CBP/p300 in interferon-gamma signaling. Proceedings of the National Academy of Sciences. 1996;**93**:15092-15096

[50] Wojciak JM, Martinez-Yamout MA, Dyson HJ, Wright PE. Structural basis for recruitment of CBP/p300 coactivators by STAT1 and STAT2 transactivation domains. The EMBO Journal. 2009;**28**:948-958

[51] Becker S, Groner B, Müller CW. Three-dimensional structure of the STAT3beta homodimer bound to DNA. Nature. 1998;**394**:145-151

[52] Mao X, Ren Z, Parker GN, Sondermann H, Pastorello MA, Wang W, et al. Structural bases of unphosphorylated STAT1 association and receptor binding. Molecular Cell. 2005;**17**:761-771

[53] Neculai D, Neculai AM, Verrier S, Straub K, Klumpp K, Pfitzner E, et al. Structure of the unphosphorylated STAT5a dimer. The Journal of Biological Chemistry. 2005;**280**:40782-40787

[54] Shuai K, Horvath CM, Huang LH, Qureshi SA, Cowburn D, Darnell JE. Interferon activation of the transcription factor Stat91 involves dimerization through SH2-phosphotyrosyl peptide interactions. Cell. 1994;**76**:821-828

[55] Haan S, Kortylewski M, Behrmann I, Müller-Esterl W, Heinrich PC, Schaper F. Cytoplasmic STAT proteins associate prior to activation. The Biochemical Journal. 2000;**345**(Pt 3):417-421

[56] Stancato LF, David M, Carter-Su C, Larner AC, Pratt WB. Preassociation of STAT1 with STAT2 and STAT3 in separate signalling complexes prior to cytokine stimulation. The Journal of Biological Chemistry. 1996;**271**:4134-4137

[57] Riebeling T, Staab J, Herrmann-Lingen C, Meyer T. DNA binding reduces the dissociation rate of STAT1 dimers and impairs the interdimeric exchange of protomers. BMC Biochemistry. 2014;**15**:28

[58] Meyer T, Gavenis K, Vinkemeier U. Cell type-specific and tyrosine phosphorylation-independent nuclear presence of STAT1 and STAT3. Experimental Cell Research. 2002;**272**:45-55

[59] Liu L, McBride KM, Reich NC. STAT3 nuclear import is independent of tyrosine phosphorylation and mediated by importin-alpha3. Proceedings of the National Academy of Sciences of the United States of America. 2005;**102**:8150-8155

[60] Yang J, Liao X, Agarwal MK, Barnes L, Auron PE, Stark GR. Unphosphorylated STAT3 accumulates in response to IL-6 and activates transcription by binding to NFkappaB. Genes & Development. 2007;**21**:1396-1408

[61] Cui X, Zhang L, Luo J, Rajasekaran A, Hazra S, Cacalano N, et al. Unphosphorylated

STAT6 contributes to constitutive cyclooxygenase-2 expression in human non-small cell lung cancer. Oncogene. 2007;**26**:4253-4260

[62] Pfeffer SR, Fan M, Du Z, Yang CH, Pfeffer LM. Unphosphorylated STAT3 regulates the antiproliferative, antiviral, and gene-inducing actions of type I interferons. Biochemical and Biophysical Research Communications. 2017;**490**:739-745

[63] Testoni B, Völlenkle C, Guerrieri F, Gerbal-Chaloin S, Blandino G, Levrero M. Chromatin dynamics of gene activation and repression in response to interferon α (IFNα) reveal new roles for phosphorylated and unphosphorylated forms of the transcription factor STAT2. The Journal of Biological Chemistry. 2011;**286**:20217-20227

[64] Yang J, Stark GR. Roles of unphosphorylated STATs in signaling. Cell Research. 2008;**18**:443-451

[65] Chatterjee-Kishore M, Wright KL, Ting JPY, Stark GR. How STAT1 mediates constitutive gene expression: A complex of unphosphorylated STAT1 and IRF1 supports transcription of the LMP2 gene. The EMBO Journal. 2000;**19**:4111-4122

[66] Min W, Pober JS, Johnson DR. Kinetically coordinated induction of TAP1 and HLA class I by IFN-gamma: The rapid induction of TAP1 by IFN-gamma is mediated by STAT1 alpha. Journal of Immunology. 1996;**156**:3174-3183

[67] Majoros A, Platanitis E, Szappanos D, Cheon H, Vogl C, Shukla P, et al. Response to interferons and antibacterial innate immunity in the absence of tyrosine-phosphorylated STAT1. EMBO Reports. 2016;**17**:367-382

[68] Lehtonen A, Matikainen S, Julkunen I. Interferons up-regulate STAT1, STAT2, and IRF family transcription factor gene expression in human peripheral blood mononuclear cells and macrophages. Journal of Immunology. 1997;**159**:794-803

[69] Decker T, Kovarik P. Serine phosphorylation of STATs. Oncogene. 2000;**19**:2628-2637

[70] Wen Z, Zhong Z, Darnell JE. Maximal activation of transcription by STAT1 and STAT3 requires both tyrosine and serine phosphorylation. Cell. 1995;**82**:241-250

[71] Wang Y, Malabarba MG, Nagy ZS, Kirken RA. Interleukin 4 regulates phosphorylation of serine 756 in the transactivation domain of STAT6. Roles for multiple phosphorylation sites and STAT6 function. The Journal of Biological Chemistry. 2004;**279**:25196-25203

[72] Varinou L, Ramsauer K, Karaghiosoff M, Kolbe T, Pfeffer K, Müller M, et al. Phosphorylation of the STAT1 transactivation domain is required for full-fledged IFN-gamma-dependent innate immunity. Immunity. 2003;**19**:793-802

[73] Morinobu A, Gadina M, Strober W, Visconti R, Fornace A, Montagna C, et al. STAT4 serine phosphorylation is critical for IL-12-induced IFN-gamma production but not for cell proliferation. Proceedings of the National Academy of Sciences of the United States of America. 2002;**99**:12281-12286

[74] Friedbichler K, Hoelbl A, Li G, Bunting KD, Sexl V, Gouilleux F, et al. Serine phosphorylation of the STAT5a C-terminus is a driving force for transformation. Frontiers in Bioscience, Landmark Edition. 2011;**16**:3043-3056

[75] Visconti R, Gadina M, Chiariello M, Chen EH, Stancato LF, Gutkind JS, et al. Importance of the MKK6/p38 pathway for interleukin-12-induced STAT4 serine phosphorylation and transcriptional activity. Blood. 2000;**96**:1844-1852

[76] Sadzak I, Schiff M, Gattermeier I, Glinitzer R, Sauer I, Saalmüller A, et al. Recruitment of STAT1 to chromatin is required for interferon-induced serine phosphorylation of STAT1 transactivation domain. Proceedings of the National Academy of Sciences of the United States of America. 2008;**105**:8944-8949

[77] Bancerek J, Poss ZC, Steinparzer I, Sedlyarov V, Pfaffenwimmer T, Mikulic I, et al. CDK8 kinase phosphorylates transcription factor STAT1 to selectively regulate the interferon response. Immunity. 2013;**38**:250-262

[78] Kovarik P, Mangold M, Ramsauer K, Heidari H, Steinborn R, Zotter A, et al. Specificity of signaling by STAT1 depends on SH2 and C-terminal domains that regulate Ser727 phosphorylation, differentially affecting specific target gene expression. The EMBO Journal. 2001;**20**:91-100

[79] Kovarik P, Stoiber D, Novy M, Decker T. STAT1 combines signals derived from IFN-gamma and LPS receptors during macrophage activation. The EMBO Journal. 1998;**17**:3660-3668

[80] Kovarik P, Stoiber D, Eyers PA, Menghini R, Neininger A, Gaestel M, et al. Stress-induced phosphorylation of STAT1 at Ser727 requires p38 mitogen-activated protein kinase whereas IFN-γ uses a different signaling pathway. Proceedings of the National Academy of Sciences of the United States of America. 1999;**96**:13956-13961

[81] Uddin S, Majchrzak B, Woodson J, Arunkumar P, Alsayed Y, Pine R, et al. Activation of the p38 mitogen-activated protein kinase by type I interferons. The Journal of Biological Chemistry. 1999;**274**:30127-30131

[82] Droescher M, Begitt A, Marg A, Zacharias M, Vinkemeier U. Cytokine-induced paracrystals prolong the activity of signal transducers and activators of transcription (STAT) and provide a model for the regulation of protein solubility by small ubiquitin-like modifier (SUMO). The Journal of Biological Chemistry. 2011;**286**:18731-18746

[83] Begitt A, Droescher M, Knobeloch KP, Vinkemeier U. SUMO conjugation of STAT1 protects cells from hyperresponsiveness to IFNγ. Blood. 2011;**118**:1002-1007

[84] Seidel HM, Milocco LH, Lamb P, Darnell JE, Stein RB, Rosen J. Spacing of palindromic half sites as a determinant of selective STAT (signal transducers and activators of transcription) DNA binding and transcriptional activity. Proceedings of the National Academy of Sciences of the United States of America. 1995;**92**:3041-3045

[85] Mikita T, Campbell D, Wu P, Williamson K, Schindler U. Requirements for interleukin-4-induced gene expression and functional characterization of STAT6. Molecular and Cellular Biology. 1996;**16**:5811-5820

[86] Koch V, Staab J, Ruppert V, Meyer T. Two glutamic acid residues in the DNA-binding domain are engaged in the release of STAT1 dimers from DNA. BMC Cell Biology. 2012;**13**:22

[87] John S, Vinkemeier U, Soldaini E, Darnell JE, Leonard WJ. The significance of tetramerization in promoter recruitment by STAT5. Molecular and Cellular Biology. 1999;**19**:1910-1918

[88] Meyer WK, Reichenbach P, Schindler U, Soldaini E, Nabholz M. Interaction of STAT5 dimers on two low affinity binding sites mediates interleukin 2 (IL-2) stimulation of IL-2 receptor alpha gene transcription. The Journal of Biological Chemistry. 1997;**272**:31821-31828

[89] Vinkemeier U, Cohen SL, Moarefi I, Chait BT, Kuriyan J, Darnell JE. DNA binding of *in vitro* activated STAT1 alpha, STAT1 beta and truncated STAT1: Interaction between NH2-terminal domains stabilizes binding of two dimers to tandem DNA sites. The EMBO Journal. 1996;**15**:5616-5626

[90] Xu X, Sun YL, Hoey T. Cooperative DNA binding and sequence-selective recognition conferred by the STAT amino-terminal domain. Science. 1996;**273**:794-797

[91] Zhang X, Darnell JE. Functional importance of STAT3 tetramerization in activation of the alpha2-macroglobulin gene. The Journal of Biological Chemistry. 2001;**276**:33576-33581

[92] Yamamoto K, Shibata F, Miyasaka N, Miura O. The human perforin gene is a direct target of STAT4 activated by IL-12 in NK cells. Biochemical and Biophysical Research Communications. 2002;**297**:1245-1252

[93] Verdier F, Rabionet R, Gouilleux F, Beisenherz-Huss C, Varlet P, Muller O, et al. A sequence of the CIS gene promoter interacts preferentially with two associated STAT5A dimers: A distinct biochemical difference between STAT5A and STAT5B. Molecular and Cellular Biology. 1998;**18**:5852-5860

[94] Hou Z, Srivastava S, Mistry MJ, Herbst MP, Bailey JP, Horseman ND. Two tandemly linked interferon-gamma-activated sequence elements in the promoter of glycosylation-dependent cell adhesion molecule 1 gene synergistically respond to prolactin in mouse mammary epithelial cells. Molecular Endocrinology. 2003;**17**:1910-1920

[95] Meyer T, Hendry L, Begitt A, John S, Vinkemeier U. A single residue modulates tyrosine dephosphorylation, oligomerization, and nuclear accumulation of STAT transcription factors. The Journal of Biological Chemistry. 2004;**279**:18998-19007

[96] Chen X, Bhandari R, Vinkemeier U, van den Akker F, Darnell JE, Kuriyan J. A reinterpretation of the dimerization interface of the N-terminal domains of STATs. Protein Science. 2003;**12**:361-365

[97] Begitt A, Droescher M, Meyer T, Schmid CD, Baker M, Antunes F, et al. STAT1-cooperative DNA binding distinguishes type 1 from type 2 interferon signaling. Nature Immunology. 2014;**15**:168-176

[98] Fujiki R, Hijikata A, Shirai T, Okada S, Kobayashi M, Ohara O. Molecular mechanism and structural basis of gain-of-function of STAT1 caused by pathogenic R274Q mutation. The Journal of Biological Chemistry. 2017;**292**:6240-6254

[99] Liu L, Okada S, Kong XF, Kreins AY, Cypowyj S, Abhyankar A, et al. Gain-of-function human STAT1 mutations impair IL-17 immunity and underlie chronic mucocutaneous candidiasis. The Journal of Experimental Medicine. 2011;**208**:1635-1648

[100] Boisson-Dupuis S, Kong XF, Okada S, Cypowyj S, Puel A, Abel L, et al. Inborn errors of human STAT1: Allelic heterogeneity governs the diversity of immunological and infectious phenotypes. Current Opinion in Immunology. 2012;**24**:364-378

[101] O'Shea JJ, Holland SM, Staudt LM. JAKs and STATs in immunity, immunodeficiency, and cancer. The New England Journal of Medicine. 2013;**368**:161-170

[102] Lorenzini T, Dotta L, Giacomelli M, Vairo D, Badolato R. STAT mutations as program switchers: Turning primary immunodeficiencies into autoimmune diseases. Journal of Leukocyte Biology. 2017;**101**:29-38

[103] Dupuis S, Jouanguy E, Al-Hajjar S, Fieschi C, Al-Mohsen IZ, Al-Jumaah S, et al. Impaired response to interferon-α/β and lethal viral disease in human STAT1 deficiency. Nature Genetics. 2003;**33**:388-391

[104] Chapgier A, Wynn RF, Jouanguy E, Filipe-Santos O, Zhang S, Feinberg J, et al. Human complete STAT1 deficiency is associated with defective type I and II IFN responses *in vitro* but immunity to some low virulence viruses *in vivo*. Journal of Immunology. 2006;**176**:5078-5083

[105] Vairo D, Tassone L, Tabellini G, Tamassia N, Gasperini S, Bazzoni F, et al. Severe impairment of IFN-γ and IFN-α responses in cells of a patient with a novel STAT1 splicing mutation. Blood. 2011;**118**:1806-1817

[106] Kristensen IA, Veirum JE, Møller BK, Christiansen M. Novel STAT1 alleles in a patient with impaired resistance to mycobacteria. Journal of Clinical Immunology. 2011;**31**:265-271

[107] Kong XF, Ciancanelli M, Al-Hajjar S, Alsina L, Zumwalt T, Bustamante J, et al. A novel form of human STAT1 deficiency impairing early but not late responses to interferons. Blood. 2010;**116**:5896-5906

[108] Dupuis S, Dargemont C, Fieschi C, Thomassin N, Rosenzweig S, Harris J, et al. Impairment of mycobacterial but not viral immunity by a germline human STAT1 mutation. Science. 2001;**293**:300-303

[109] Chapgier A, Boisson-Dupuis S, Jouanguy E, Vogt G, Feinberg J, Prochnicka-Chalufour A, et al. Novel STAT1 alleles in otherwise healthy patients with mycobacterial disease. PLoS Genetics. 2006;**2**:1193-1206

[110] Takezaki S, Yamada M, Kato M, Park MJ, Maruyama K, Yamazaki Y, et al. Chronic mucocutaneous candidiasis caused by a gain-of-function mutation in the STAT1 DNA-binding domain. Journal of Immunology. 2012;**189**:1521-1526

[111] van de Veerdonk FL, Plantinga TS, Hoischen A, Smeekens SP, Joosten LA, Gilissen C, et al. STAT1 mutations in autosomal dominant chronic mucocutaneous candidiasis. The New England Journal of Medicine. 2011;**365**:54-61

[112] Hijikata A, Tsuji T, Shionyu M, Shirai T. Decoding disease-causing mechanisms of missense mutations from supramolecular structures. Scientific Reports. 2017;**7**:8541

[113] Staab J, Herrmann-Lingen C, Meyer T. Clinically relevant dimer interface mutants of STAT1 transcription factor exhibit differential gene expression. PLoS One. 2013;**8**:e69903

[114] Sampaio EP, Hsu AP, Pechacek J, Bax HI, Dias DL, Paulson ML, et al. Signal transducer and activator of transcription 1 (STAT1) gain-of-function mutations and disseminated coccidioidomycosis and histoplasmosis. The Journal of Allergy and Clinical Immunology. 2013;**131**:1624-1634

[115] Uzel G, Sampaio EP, Lawrence MG, Hsu AP, Hackett M, Dorsey MJ, et al. Dominant gain-of-function STAT1 mutations in FOXP3 wild-type immune dysregulation-polyendocrinopathy-enteropathy-X-linked-like syndrome. The Journal of Allergy and Clinical Immunology. 2013;**131**:1611-1623

[116] Ueki M, Yamada M, Ito K, Tozawa Y, Morino S, Horikoshi Y, et al. A heterozygous dominant-negative mutation in the coiled-coil domain of STAT1 is the cause of autosomal-dominant Mendelian susceptibility to mycobacterial diseases. Clinical Immunology. 2017;**174**:24-31

Chapter 4

Distinct E2F-Mediated Transcriptional Mechanisms in Cell Proliferation, Endoreplication and Apoptosis

Hideyuki Komori, Ritsuko Iwanaga, Andrew P. Bradford, Keigo Araki and Kiyoshi Ohtani

Abstract

E2F and DP family proteins are evolutionally conserved transcription factors among higher eukaryotes. E2F and DP proteins typically form a heterodimeric complex, which controls cell proliferation by regulating expression of growth-related genes. In addition, E2F family proteins have roles in various cellular events that require the expression of context-specific genes. E2F proteins use distinct mechanisms to regulate context-specific genes in different circumstances. The primary goal of this chapter is to compare three distinct mechanisms of mammalian E2F-mediated transcriptional regulation that control cell proliferation, endoreplication and apoptosis. Briefly, E2F7 and E2F8 control endoreplication by suppressing the expression of their target genes. They do not require DP or pRb. In control of apoptosis, E2F1 regulates the expression of the tumor suppressor gene *Arf* by binding to a non-canonical E2F binding site, within the *Arf* promoter, in a DP-independent manner. Furthermore, we examine the functions of E2F and DP in *Drosophila melanogaster* (fruit fly) to identify those mechanisms of E2F-mediated transcriptional regulation that have been evolutionarily conserved. The detailed mechanisms of how E2F protein regulates the expression of context-specific target genes will be instrumental in understanding how a single family of transcription factor regulates diverse pleiotropic cellular processes in an organism.

Keywords: E2F, DP, pRb, Arf, p53, cell cycle, endoreplication, apoptosis

1. Introduction

The temporal control of gene expression is essential to the execution of cellular events such as proliferation, growth, self-renewal, differentiation and death. For example, a proliferating cell performs the sequential processes of the cell cycle by the orderly expression of genes involved in DNA replication, DNA repair, mitosis and cytokinesis [1, 2]. During the cell cycle, *E2* promoter binding *f*actor (E2F) and *D*RTF1-*p*olypeptide (DP) form a heterodimeric complex E2F/DP, which functions with retinoblastoma protein (pRb) to regulate the timing of expression of growth-related genes at the level of transcription [1–5]. In quiescent cells, the E2F/DP complexes interact with pRb family proteins to prevent cell cycle re-entry by actively repressing the expression of growth-related genes (**Figure 1A** and **B**). Mitogenic signals promote the assembly and activation of the Cyclin D/cyclin-dependent kinase (cdk) 4 complex in the cell nucleus. Phosphorylation of pRb family proteins by the Cyclin D-cdk4 complex results in their dissociation from the E2F/DP complex (**Figure 1A**), and consequently growth-related genes are de-repressed. The free E2F/DP complexes also promote transcription of their target genes (**Figure 1A** and **B**). Primary E2F target genes in the cell cycle encode DNA-replication factors. In addition, the E2F/DP complex induces the expression of cyclins (E, A, and B) and genes involved in DNA repair, mitosis and cytokinesis. Thus, the pRb/E2F/DP pathway controls not only the G1/S transition, but also influences other processes of the cell cycle. Once the level of mitogen signals is reduced, cdk activity is down-regulated, under-phosphorylated pRb family proteins accumulate, E2F activity is repressed, and cells exit from the cell cycle.

Genome wide gene expression profiles and analysis of the function of individual E2F family proteins have revealed that E2F family members have roles in various cellular processes including endoreplication [6], cell death [7], autophagy [8] and differentiation [9]. Since it is unlikely that E2F simultaneously induces genes involved in these distinct, often mutually exclusive cellular processes, cells must have multiple mechanisms, by which specific E2F target genes are expressed to function in line with intracellular circumstances. Indeed, the mechanism of E2F1 regulation of tumor suppressor genes, *Alternative reading frame of cdkn2a* (*Arf*), *p27* and *p73* is distinct from that of growth-related genes [10–12]. Surprisingly, the requirement for DP is different between E2F1 regulation of *Arf* and growth-related genes such as *cell division cycle 6* (*cdc6*), implying that DP protein is not involved in all E2F-mediated transcriptional regulation [13]. In this chapter, we describe mechanisms of E2F-mediated transcriptional regulation in three different cellular functions, cell proliferation, endoreplication and apoptosis, and discuss the requirement for DP in these processes. In addition, we compare and contrast these mechanisms in mammals and flies, to identify those that have been conserved or emerged during the process of evolution.

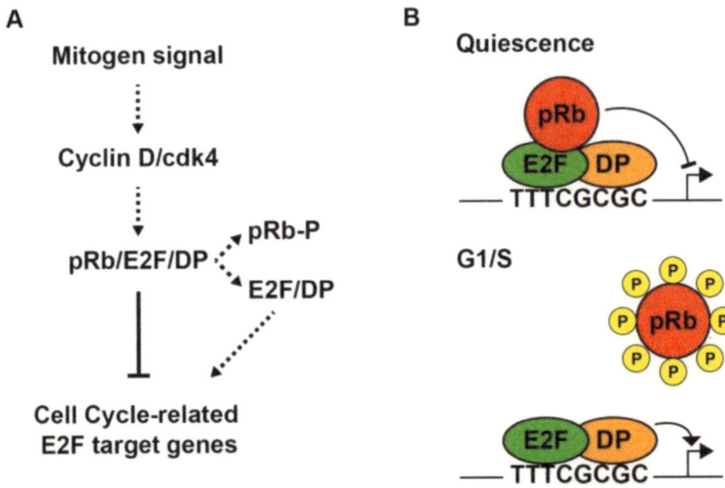

Figure 1.
The E2F/DP complex controls cell cycle progression with pRB. (A) Schematic view of the pRb/E2F/DP pathway. Solid line indicates the function of pRb/E2F/DP complex to repress the expression of growth-related E2F-target genes in quiescence. Dashed arrows indicate the signal cascade following activation by mitogenic signals. pRb-P indicates phosphorylated pRb. (B) Regulation of growth-related E2F target genes by the pRB/E2F/DP complex during the cell cycle. The pRb/E2F/DP complex actively represses the transcription of growth-related E2F target genes in quiescence, while free activator E2F/DP complex promotes transcription of the target genes when pRb family proteins are phosphorylated by G1-cyclin/cdk.

2. Structures of mammalian and fly E2F and DP family members

The human and mouse genomes contain eight E2F family genes and three DP family genes (**Figure 2**) [3]. E2F family proteins can be distinguished as "activator" or "repressor" by their functions in transcription, or "typical" or "atypical" based on their structure. E2F1–5 genes encode proteins composed of a winged-helix *D*NA-*b*inding *d*omain (DBD), *L*eucine *z*ipper (LZ) domain, *M*arked-*b*ox (MB) domain and *t*rans*a*ctivation *d*omain (TAD) that includes pRb-binding motif (**Figure 2**). E2F6 protein lacks the TAD and pRb-binding motif (**Figure 2**). E2F1–3a are categorized as activator E2Fs because they are essential to activate transcription of target genes in cell culture [3]. E2F3b-5 are designated repressor E2Fs since their main function is to suppress the expression of target genes by interacting with pRb family proteins in resting states [14–16]. E2F6 is also a repressor E2F, but functions without interacting pRb family proteins [17–19]. E2F1–6 proteins interact with one of the DP proteins through LZ and MB domains (dimerization domain: DD). All DP family members possess a DBD and DD [3]. In addition, the C-terminus of DP1 can interact with TFIIH, suggesting that DP1 directly contributes to activation of target gene transcription [20]. DP1 and DP2 support the transcriptional activation of E2F target genes while DP3 functions to inhibit E2F-dependent transcription [21, 22]. The E2F/DP complex typically recognizes specific DNA sequences $TTT^{C}/_{G}{}^{G}/_{C}CG^{C}/_{G}$ (hereafter referred to as "canonical E2F binding site" in this chapter) [23]. E2F1 is also able to

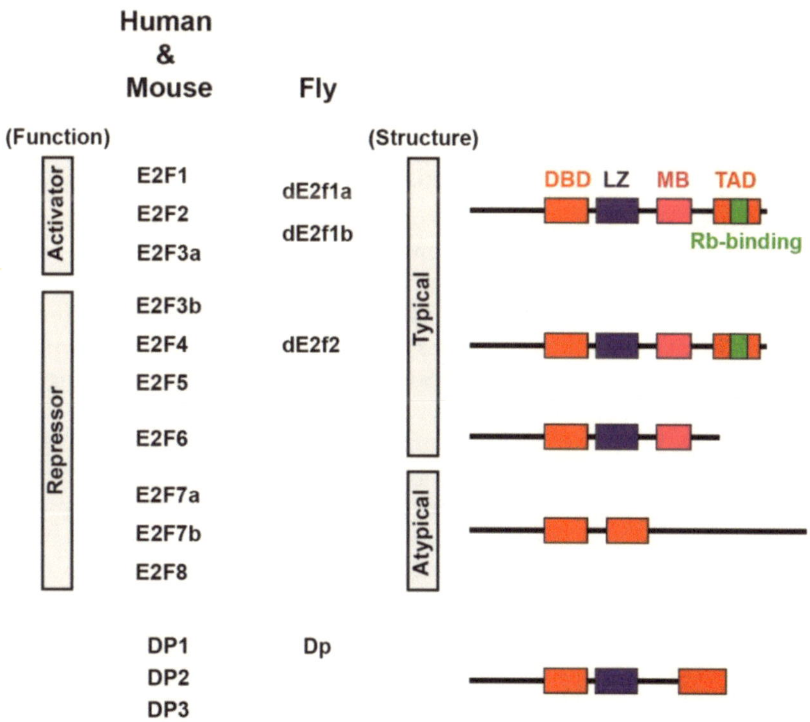

Figure 2.
E2F and DP family members in human, mouse and fly. E2F families can be divided into two groups by functional or structural properties. Activator E2Fs are required to induce expression of growth-related E2F target genes at G1/S phase transition. E2F3a-5 are expressed in quiescence (G0) and G1 phase to repress target gene transcription by pRb-dependent mechanisms. E2F6–8 have the ability to repress target gene transcription by pRb-independent mechanisms. Typical E2Fs possess DBD, LZ, MB and TAD, while atypical E2Fs possess two DBD without a TAD. DP family proteins share DBD and LZ. TAD is found in mammalian DP1.

bind to a non-canonical E2F binding site called *E*2F-*r*esponsive *e*lement of *A*rf (EREA), comprised of the sequence CGCGCGCGCGCCTCC [10].

After completion of the human and mouse genome sequencing projects, searches for homologous sequences to the E2F-DBD identified atypical E2F family members, E2F7 and E2F8 that are structurally distinct from E2F1 to 6 (**Figure 2**) [24–29]. E2F7 and 8 contain two DBDs but lack a transactivation domain. These atypical E2Fs recognize canonical E2F binding sites in a DP-independent manner and function to repress transcription of E2F target genes by a pRb-independent mechanism.

The fly genome contains two *e2f* genes and a single *dp* gene [3, 4, 30]. *de2f1* encodes two isoforms, which function as transcriptional activators, while dE2f2 acts as a repressor in transcription (**Figure 2**) [31, 32]. Because all other higher eukaryotes also possess functional homolog of activator E2F, repressor E2F and DP, the mechanism of transcriptional control by the E2F/DP complex has been evolutionally conserved [33]. Atypical E2Fs are shared in several model organisms including mammals, worm and plant, but not in fly (**Figure 2**) [33]. DP-independent transcriptional regulation by atypical E2Fs seems to have been emerged and been lost during the process of evolution.

3. The role of the E2F/DP complex in cell proliferation

3.1 DP is essential in transcriptional regulation of growth-related E2F target genes in cultured cells

The concept of the pRb/E2F/DP pathway is based primarily on evidence obtained using rodent fibroblasts in culture [1–5]. The advantage of this system is the ease of manipulating the proliferative capacity of cells without losing cell viability by the absence or presence of fetal bovine serum in the culture medium [34, 35]. Fibroblasts continuously proliferate in culture medium that contains abundant serum. Withdrawing serum from the media causes cells to exit from the cell cycle, while re-introduction of serum leads to re-entry into the cell cycle. Thus, this system enables control of endogenous E2F activity by manipulating the amount of serum in culture media. In addition, using expression vectors and recombinant adenovirus containing various E2F genes, we can examine the specific activity of individual E2F proteins in quiescent fibroblast without other confounding proliferating signals [2]. The functional analysis of individual E2F proteins in quiescent fibroblasts revealed that activator E2Fs are sufficient to promote the G1/S transition in the cell cycle [34, 35]. Conversely, loss of activator E2Fs causes cell cycle arrest at G1 phase [36]. Accordingly, DP1 is required for G1/S transition and cell proliferation in human fibroblasts [13]. These observations indicate that the activator E2F/DP complexes promote and regulate the G1/S transition in cultured cells. However, subsequent studies revealed that the cell cycle arrest caused by concomitant loss of activator E2Fs in cultured fibroblasts is mediated through the p53-p21 axis, which reduces cdk activity [37]. Inactivation of p53 restores the proliferative ability of *E2f1–3* triple mutant fibroblasts [38]. These results suggest that cells have permissive factor(s), which promote G1/S transition in the absence of activator E2Fs, and raise the question of how activator E2Fs suppress p53 activity in proliferating cells. A strong candidate of E2F target genes that induce activation of p53 in this context was *Arf*, since permanent loss of *E2f3* induces *Arf* expression [38, 39]. However, acute inactivation of E2F activators does not increase *Arf* expression and activation of p53 does not require *Arf* in *E2f1–3* triple mutant fibroblasts [38]. Therefore, induction of *Arf* gene expression by loss of *E2f3* is presumably an indirect effect and activator E2Fs suppress activation of p53 by Arf-independent mechanisms in fibroblasts. Elucidating the mechanisms, by which activator E2Fs suppress p53 activity in proliferating cells, will provide deeper understanding of how activator E2Fs regulate cell proliferation.

Cell culture systems and *in vitro* biochemical experiments have also revealed molecular mechanisms underlying transcriptional regulation of target genes by the E2F/DP complex [1, 2, 5]. Expression levels of growth-related E2F target genes are very low in quiescent fibroblasts, while serum stimulation increases the expression of these genes concomitant with phosphorylation of pRb family proteins by G1-cyclin/cdks [1–5]. Indeed, loss of all *Rb* family genes increases the level of growth-related E2F target gene expression in quiescent mouse fibroblasts [40]. The concept that pRb/E2F/DP complex actively represses the transcription of growth-related E2F target genes in quiescence was conceived based on results from reporter assays, in which the promoter region of an E2F target gene is isolated and fused upstream of a reporter gene such as *chloramphenicol acetyltransferase* or *luciferase* to monitor promoter activity [34, 41]. Analysis of such reporter activity during the cell cycle revealed that the wild-type promoter recapitulates endogenous gene expression patterns throughout the cell cycle, while mutations in canonical E2F binding sites de-represses the promoter activity in quiescence and does not allow further up-regulation at the G1/S transition (**Figure 3**). E2F4 and p130 occupied canonical E2F binding sites on promoters of growth-related E2F target genes in quiescence [14, 16]. DP1 is required for E2F4 binding on the promoter of *cdc6* in quiescent human fibroblasts and for repression of the *cdc6* promoter activity [13] (Komori & Ohtani unpublished data). pRb family proteins repress E2F target promoter activity by recruiting histone modifier proteins and chromatin remodeling complexes [42–47]. Thus, the repressor E2F/DP complex acts as a platform on the target promoters to recruit pRb family proteins, which induce a dynamic change of chromatin structure, robustly shutting down the transcription of growth-related E2F target genes (**Figure 1B**).

Activator E2Fs induce stronger activation of E2F target gene transcription compared to repressor E2Fs in reporter assays. Co-overexpression of DPs induces further activation of reporter transcription while knockdown of DP1 reduces promoter activity induced by activator E2Fs [13, 48, 49]. Thus, DP is essential for both active repression and activation of growth-related E2F target gene transcription

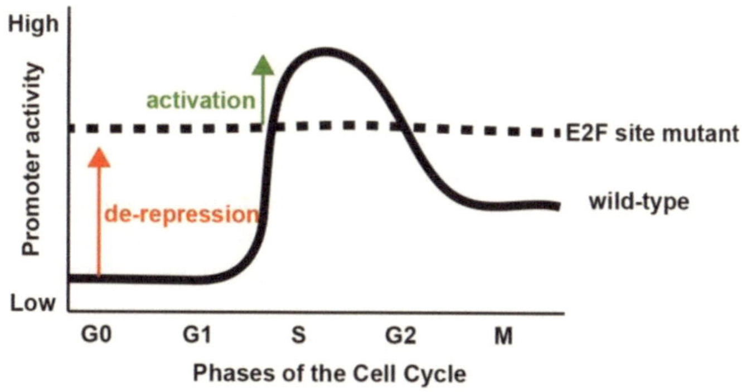

Figure 3.
The promoter activity of growth-related E2F target genes during the cell cycle. Solid line indicates the activity of wild-type promoter of growth-related E2F target genes. Dashed line indicates the activity of canonical E2F binding site mutant promoter of growth-related E2F target genes. The difference in promoter activity between wild-type and E2F binding site mutant is due to pRB/E2F/DP complex-dependent repression. Activator E2Fs increase the wild-type promoter activity to a higher level than the mutant promoter activity at the G1/S phase transition.

(**Figure 1B**). The main role of DP in the regulation of growth-related E2F target gene expression is in DNA binding of the E2F/DP complex [3, 20]. A monomer of E2F or DP is able to bind to DNA *in vitro*, whereas the heterodimer complex shows much stronger DNA binding affinity [48, 49]. Structural analysis of the complex of E2F4/DP2 bound to a canonical E2F binding site revealed that the E2F/DP complex holds DNA by DBDs of both E2F and DP [50]. Thus, DP protein ensures a stable binding of the E2F/DP complex to precisely control expression of growth-related E2F target genes during the cell cycle.

3.2 The role of the E2F/DP complex in mouse development

In order to form functional tissues and organs, stem cells and progenitor cells continuously proliferate to generate progeny cells, which must exit from the cell cycle at the onset of commitment to a differentiated state [51]. Because loss of all activator E2Fs or loss of DP1 induces cell cycle arrest of cells in culture [13, 36, 52], *E2f1–3* triple mutant was expected to show a premature exhaustion of cell proliferation during development. However, the *E2f1–3* triple mutant mouse embryo grows to mid-gestation stage without severe defects of cell proliferation [53, 54]. In the absence of activator E2Fs, the Myc family transcription factors compensate for their function to promote the G1/S transition [54, 55]. n-Myc can functionally substitute for activator E2Fs in retinal progenitors, while c-Myc complements activator E2Fs in intestinal stem cells. *E2f1–3* triple mutant embryos also exhibit an apoptotic phenotype in multiple tissues, in which activation of p53 is observed. This suggests that activator E2Fs suppress the activation of p53 during development *in vivo*, in addition to cells in culture. *E2f1–3* triple knock out analysis revealed another aspect of the function of activator E2Fs [55]. The expression of growth-related E2F target genes is increased by inactivation of E2f1–3 in differentiated cells while loss of E2F1–3 reduces the expression of growth-related E2F target genes in proliferating progenitor cells, suggesting that E2F1–3 contribute to repress target gene expression in differentiated cells. However, loss of E2F1–3 does not induce differentiated cells to re-enter into the cell cycle, implying that, in addition to de-repression of growth-related E2F target genes, other factors are required to cause re-entry of terminally differentiated cells into the cell cycle.

Removing all E2f genes from a single mouse is technically impossible at this stage. The DP family has three members and DP1 is highly expressed in many tissues. Thus, it is anticipated that loss of DP1 would mimic the phenotype expected due to elimination of all E2F/DP complexes in the mouse. *DP1* mutant mice die *in utero* due to defects in placenta development, while their somatic cells proliferate without severe defects [56, 57]. There is a possibility that other DP family proteins complement the function of DP1 in *DP1* mutant animals. However, the levels of DP2 expression are very low in the wild-type and its expression is not significantly changed in *DP1* mutant embryos. The expression of DP3 has not been investigated in *DP1* mutant mice. However, since DP3 inhibits activation of growth-related target genes by E2F1 in cultured cells [21, 22], it is not likely that DP3 compensates for DP1 function. In conclusion, the E2F/DP complex function is required for normal development, but the viability seems to be determined by functions that are independent from cell cycle control.

3.3 The role of DP in fly development

Mammalian genomes contain several E2F and DP family members, and their functional relationships are very complicated. Because the fly genome contains two E2Fs, only one DP and no atypical E2Fs, the combinatorial interactions and possibility of compensation by other family members are more limited [4, 33]. In drosophila, loss of *de2f1* reduces cell proliferation during development [58]. The decline in cell proliferation induced by loss of *de2f1* is restored by removing *de2f2* gene function, indicating that dE2f1 and dE2f2 have opposite functions in control of cell proliferation [31, 32]. *dDP* mutant larvae phenocopy the *de2f1 and de2f2* double mutant with respect to cell proliferation and lethality at the late pupal stage [31, 32]. The viability of the *dDP* mutant fly is rescued by restoring the defects in muscle development and/or fat body cell growth [59, 60], implying that the lethality is due to non-cell cycle function of dDP. These indicate that the E2F/DP complexes are not necessary for cell proliferation during fly development. The possibility that dMyc may compensate for the function of the dE2f/dDP complex in cell proliferation has yet to be examined.

4. The role of atypical E2Fs in endoreplication

4.1 Atypical E2Fs inhibit cell cycle progression in cultured cell

E2F7 and E2F8 are atypical E2F proteins, which are composed of two DBDs lacking a transactivation domain or pRb binding motif (**Figure 2**) [3, 24–29, 33]. They do not interact with DP, and thus atypical E2Fs function independently of DP protein. Since overexpression of atypical E2Fs represses the promoter activity of growth-related E2F target genes, they are designated repressor E2Fs. They function via a pRb-independent mechanism. E2F7 recruits the transcriptional co-repressor CtBP to repress the activity of its target promoter in fibroblasts [61]. Details of molecular mechanisms of how atypical E2Fs regulate E2F target genes have been controversial. DBD1 of E2F7 is similar to the DBD of the E2F family, while DBD2 of E2F7 is homologous to that of the DP family. Both DBDs are necessary for the DNA binding ability of atypical E2Fs. Crystal structure analysis revealed that DBD1 and DBD2 bind to a typical E2F binding site in a manner similar to the E2F4/DP2 heterodimeric complex [62]. This suggests the possibility that atypical E2Fs are able to function as a monomer (**Figure 4A**). However, they form a homodimer or a heterodimer of E2F7 and E2F8 in cells (**Figure 4A**) [24–29]. How this dimeric complex of atypical E2Fs binds to DNA remains to be addressed. In addition, it is reported that E2F7 inhibits the function of E2F1 by direct interaction (**Figure 4A**) [61]. How then does an E2F1/E2F7 heterodimer bind to DNA and how does E2F7 dominate E2F1 activity on their target promoter? Overexpression of atypical E2Fs inhibits proliferation of fibroblasts in culture [24–29]. Expression of atypical E2Fs is upregulated in G1/S transition of fibroblasts because their expression is under the control of typical E2Fs. These suggest that atypical E2Fs may function as a negative feedback loop to antagonize the function of activator E2Fs in S-phase of the cell cycle. However, cells can proliferate in the presence of atypical E2Fs. If they are dispensable in the control of cell proliferation, what is the role of atypical E2Fs in the physiological setting?

4.2 Atypical E2Fs control endoreplication during mouse development

Mouse atypical E2Fs play crucial roles in endoreplication of placental *t*rophoblast*g*iant *c*ells (TGCs) and liver hepatocytes [3, 33, 63]. While the archetypal cell cycle proceeds to G2 and M phases after completing DNA replication, endoreplication is a variant cell cycle, which repeats the cycle of G1 and S phase in the absence of intervening mitoses (**Figure 4B**) [64]. Consequently, endoreplication produces mononucleated polyploid cells. Since endoreplication does not permit cells to enter

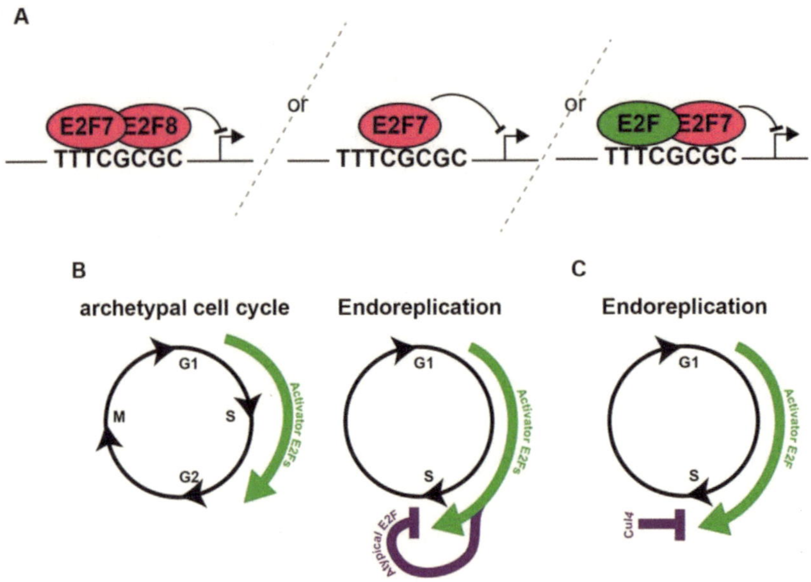

Figure 4.
Atypical E2Fs regulate growth-related E2F target genes by DP-independent mechanism(s) and control endoreplication. (A) Possible mechanisms to repress target promoters by atypical E2Fs. Atypical E2Fs repress the transcription of their target genes by forming a dimer of atypical E2Fs, or monomer, or binding to an activator E2F. (B) Archetypal cell cycle and endoreplication. Four phases (G1, S, G2, M) are proceeded in the archetypal cell cycle, while endoreplication repeats G1 and S phases. Atypical E2Fs are induced at G1/S phase and antagonize activator E2Fs at S phase in an endoreplication cycle. (C) Endoreplication in fly. Cul4 induces an acute degradation of dE2f1 to skip G2 and M phases.

into mitosis, precise control of mitotic cyclin/cdk activity is important to determine the initiation and termination of endoreplication.

Loss of *E2f1–3* genes results in continuous excess rounds of endoreplication in TGCs, while double knock out of *E2f7* and *E2f8* genes induces a defect in endoreplication [3, 63]. Thus, the activator E2F/DP complex promotes exit from endoreplication, while atypical E2Fs maintain it. The reduced number of endoreplication cycles in *E2f7* and *E2f8* double mutant TGCs is partially restored by eliminating the function of *E2f1*. These results indicate that DP-independent E2F regulation by atypical E2Fs competitively antagonizes the function of DP-dependent E2F regulation by typical E2Fs during endoreplication (**Figure 4B**). Atypical E2Fs suppresses the expression of Cyclin A as well as cdc2, preventing the entry into M phase during endoreplication. The transient up-regulation of atypical E2F expression during S phase is important to suppress the expression of target genes immediately after DNA replication [24–29]. However, the transient accumulation of atypical E2Fs does not instruct the timing of initiation and termination of endoreplication. The basal level of their expression is changed during tissue development [63]. An increase in the basal level of atypical E2Fs expression allows cells to initiate endoreplication, while a reduction in basal levels of atypical E2Fs induces cells to exit from endoreplication. Thus, a combination of developmental and cell cycle cues determines the timing and duration of endoreplication during tissue development.

4.3 Endoreplication in fly development

Fly is a model organism that lacks atypical *E2f* genes in its genome [4, 33]. Yet, endoreplication is conducted in cells of multiple tissues including secretory cells of salivary glands, subperineural glia of the brain, and ovarian nurse and follicle cells [64]. How is cdk activity downregulated immediately after DNA replication in these cell types without atypical E2Fs? Instead of atypical E2F-mediated suppression of E2F target gene expression, ubiquitin ligase Cul4 induces a rapid degradation of dE2f1 during S phase, reducing the expression of E2F target genes including Cyclin E and mitotic cyclins (**Figure 4C**) [65]. Downregulation of Cyclin E/cdk2 activity during S phase does not allow cell cycle to progress through the G2/M phase transition in fly, thereby returning the cell cycle back into G1 phase, resulting in endoreplication [66, 67]. These observations imply that organisms lacking atypical E2Fs have mechanism(s) to complement their function.

5. The role of E2F1 in apoptosis and tumor suppression

5.1 E2F1 induces apoptosis in a DP-independent manner in mammalian fibroblasts

Cultured cell systems also demonstrated that E2F1 can function to induce apoptosis [1, 2, 7]. Overexpression of E2F1 induces p53-dependent and p53-dependent apoptosis in cultured cells in the absence of survival signals provided by serum (**Figure 5A**). Overexpression of E2F1 induces the expression of Arf, which activates p53 through suppression of MDM2 [1, 2, 5, 10, 68]. E2F1 bypasses p53-dependent apoptosis by inducing the expression of the p53 homolog, p73 [69, 70]. In contrast to control of cell proliferation, DP1 and DP2 are not necessary for E2F1-induced apoptosis [13], indicating that E2F1-induced apoptosis is the second model of DP-independent E2F function. The function of E2F1 to induce apoptosis is intuitively contradictory to its role in promoting cell proliferation. Why does E2F1 protein have these opposing roles? Since endogenous pRb family proteins are unable to suppress the activity of E2F generated by overproduction of E2F, exogenous overexpression of E2F1 is supposed to recapitulate deregulated E2F activity that results from functional defects in pRb family proteins. Consistent with this theory, adenovirus E1A protein, which directly binds to pRb and inhibits its function, also induces apoptosis through the Arf-MDM2-p53 pathway in fibroblasts [71–73]. Therefore, the role of E2F1-mediated apoptosis has been interpreted as a defensive mechanism to protect against and/or counter oncogenic activation of E2F1 that induces abnormal proliferation in the context of pRb dysfunction.

5.2 DP-independent regulation of Arf expression by E2F1 in mammalian fibroblast

The transcription of the *Arf* and *p73* genes is not increased by endogenous E2F activated by serum stimulation in fibroblasts, while the expression of growth-related E2F target genes is induced (**Figure 5B**) [10, 12]. One possible explanation of the inability of endogenously activated E2F to increase *Arf* and *p73* expression is that serum stimulation activates survival signals that specifically counteract the induction of apoptotic genes by E2F [74]. Phosphatidylinositol-3 kinase (PI3K) signaling inhibits expression of some apoptotic genes, induced by overexpression of E2F1, such as AMPKa2, which is involved in metabolism and is not a typical apoptotic gene [75]. However, it is not clear whether the PI3K signaling regulates these genes at the transcriptional level or post-transcriptional level. In addition, PI3K signaling does not suppress the induction of *Arf* gene expression by overexpression of E2F1 [76]. Therefore, mechanisms must exist to allow the *Arf* gene to specifically sense and respond to deregulated E2F activity.

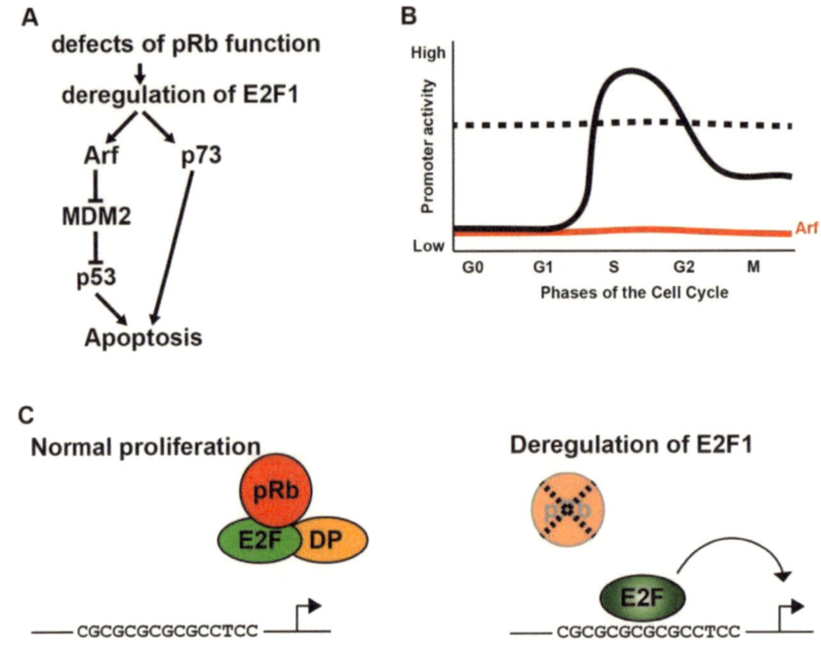

Figure 5.
E2F1 regulation of Arf gene transcription and apoptosis in Rb-deficiency. (A) Schematic view of E2F1-induced apoptosis. E2F1 induces apoptosis through p53-dependent and -independent mechanisms. (B) Arf promoter activity during the cell cycle. Black line indicates the activity of the wild-type promoter of growth-related E2F target genes. Dashed black line indicates the activity of canonical E2F binding site mutant promoter in growth-related E2F target genes. Red line indicates the activity of the Arf promoter. (C) E2F regulation of the Arf promoter in normal cell proliferation and in the context of deregulated E2F activity in response to dysfunction of pRb.

We have approached this issue by investigating mechanisms of how E2F regulates *Arf* gene expression in human fibroblast [10, 13]. Analysis of *Arf* promoter regulation has revealed the following points. (i) the pRb/E2F/DP complex does not actively suppress the *Arf* promoter during the cell cycle (**Figure 5C**). (ii) The *Arf* promoter is very sensitive to deregulated E2F activity, but not to E2F activity induced by serum stimulation. (iii) E2F1 regulation of the *Arf* promoter does not require DP. (iv) The regulation is mediated through a non-canonical E2F binding site, EREA (**Figure 5C**). The sequence of EREA is highly conserved in the *Arf* promoters in human and mouse and an isolated EREA reporter construct from the mouse *Arf* promoter showed similar activity in response to serum stimulation and overexpression of E2F1. Thus, E2F regulation of EREA may be shared between mouse and human [10]. Our finding raised a new question of how E2F1 binds to EREA. *In vitro* studies showed that, while E2F1 alone is able to bind to a canonical E2F binding site, the presence of DP1 drastically enhances E2F1 binding affinity to this DNA element. In contrast, the presence of DP does not impact E2F1 binding to EREA. Since the presence of DP does not interfere with E2F1 binding to the EREA, the E2F/DP complex perhaps binds to EREA utilizing only the E2F DBD. In general, a transcription factor works in combination or acts synergistically with a functional partner protein. Thus, there may be specific factor(s) that cooperatively function with E2F1 to regulate EREA.

In parallel to our study, Hallstrom et al. reported different mechanisms of regulation of E2F1-induced apoptosis [74, 77]. They found that (i) The MB domain determines specificity of E2F1 to induce apoptosis. A chimeric E2F1 mutant containing E2F3 MB loses the ability to induce apoptosis, while insertion of the E2F1 MB domain into E2F3 confers the ability to induce apoptosis. (ii) E2F1 binds to Jab1, a subunit of the COP9 signalosome (CSN), through its MB domain. The E2F1-Jab1 interaction is specific to E2F1 because the amino acid sequence of MB domain varies among individual E2F proteins. (iii) Jab1 enhances E2F1-indued activation of p53 and apoptosis. (iv) Jab1 enhances induction of *Arf* gene expression by overexpression of E2F1. (v) Jab1 binds to the *Arf* promoter [78]. These are indirect evidence, but suggest that Jab1 contributes to activation of *Arf* gene transcription by E2F1, leading us to postulate that the EREA plays a role in Jab1 binding to the *Arf* promoter. Further investigation will be required to reveal details of mechanisms underlying E2F regulation of *Arf* gene expression and apoptosis.

5.3 Arf suppresses tumorigenesis in the Rb mutant mouse

Homozygous mutation of the *Rb* gene induces ectopic proliferation and apoptosis in multiple tissues of mouse embryos [3, 79]. These phenotypes are rescued by removing *E2f1* gene function [80], suggesting that pRb regulates E2F activity and deregulated E2F1 induces apoptosis *in vivo*. Ablation of the *Arf* gene does not suppress the apoptotic phenotype in *Rb* homozygous mutant embryos [81], indicating that E2F1 induces apoptosis through Arf-independent mechanisms in particular cell types. The *Rb* gene is one of the most prominent tumor suppressor genes and loss of pRb function is observed in wide variety of human cancers [5]. Heterozygous mutation predicts retinoblastoma and osteoblastoma in human [5]. These observations suggest that E2F1-induced *Arf* may counteract tumorigenesis in *Rb* mutant cells. In a mouse model, heterozygous mutation of *Rb* typically produced pituitary and thyroid tumors, which is used in study of tumor suppressive function of *Rb in vivo* [79]. In these tumors, wild-type *Rb* allele is also lost during tumor formation and loss of *E2f1* suppresses tumorigenesis in heterozygous *Rb* mutant mice [82], indicating that E2F1 is deregulated to induce abnormal proliferation in these tumor cells. In addition, because the tumor phenotype in pituitary and thyroid of *Rb* heterozygous mutant mouse is exacerbated by loss of *Arf* [81], it is likely that deregulated E2F1 activity counteracts tumor formation through inducing *Arf* in these tumors. $Rb^{-/+}$; $Arf^{-/-}$ compound mutant mice develop pituitary gland lesions earlier than $Rb^{-/+}$ and $Rb^{-/+}$; $p53^{-/-}$ [81]. Therefore, Arf should function independently of p53 to suppress tumor formation in the pituitary and thyroid glands of *Rb* mutant mice.

5.4 E2F-induced apoptosis in fly requires DP

Overexpression of *de2f1* or homozygous mutation of *rbf1* induces apoptosis in multiple tissues in the fly [4, 83], indicating that consistent with vertebrates, deregulation of dE2f1 induces cell death in fly. However, there are two inconsistent observations. Firstly, dE2f1 requires dDP to induce apoptosis [4, 84, 85]. Secondly, dE2f1-induced apoptosis is primarily independent of p53 [86]. The role of fly p53 in apoptosis is not as predominant as that of mammalian p53 and the *Arf* gene does not exist in the fly genome. Mechanisms of both E2F1-induced and p53-dependent apoptosis, and interactions between them, may have been modified and adapted during the process of evolution.

6. Conclusion and perspective

In this chapter, we considered multiple roles of E2F transcription factor by introducing three distinct mechanisms of E2F-mediated transcription. The classic model of the E2F/DP complex explains how the heterodimeric complex regulates growth-related E2F target genes by collaborating with pRb family proteins during the cell cycle [1–5]. There is no doubt that the pRb/E2F/DP pathway instructs both entry into and exit from the cell cycle. However, recent studies revealed that cells have complementary mechanisms in control of cell cycle progression at the G1/S phase transition. Future studies should address the mechanisms, by which cells can control the exit from the cell cycle in the absence of the pRB/E2F/DP complex. The classic E2F/DP model is not sufficient to explain all function of E2F family proteins. Two additional mechanisms, described above, at least partly fill that knowledge gap. Atypical E2Fs play a crucial role in endoreplication by antagonizing the function of activator E2Fs in DP-independent and Rb-independent manners [3, 33, 63]. In addition to their role in endoreplication, atypical E2Fs may also mediate tumor suppression in multiple tissues including liver and skin [87, 88]. How they function in suppressing tumorigenesis is an important question for future studies. E2F1 also functions via DP-independent mechanisms, which mediate tumor suppression via regulation of apoptotic genes including *Arf* [13]. In addition to modulating tumor suppression, these E2F1 pathways may have a role in restricting the plasticity of cell fate in differentiated cells. Overexpression of four transcription factors (Oct4, Sox2, c-Myc and klf4) reverts the competence of fibroblast to the level of pluripotent embryonic stem cells [89]. The efficiency of this reprograming is restricted by the pRb-p53 pathway [90, 91]. E2F-dependent transcription of *Arf*, or regulation of p53, may be involved in the mechanism to restrict the plasticity of cell fate in fibroblasts. In addition, *Rb* and *Arf* contribute to limit the reversion of myocytes to myoblasts in regeneration of muscle [92]. These possibilities merit further investigation, and discoveries of new mechanisms of E2F regulation of its target genes will open a new paradigm to understand the diverse roles of E2F transcription factor families.

Acknowledgements

This work was supported in part by JSPS KAKENHI Grant Number JP15K06957.

Conflict of interest

Authors have no conflict of interest.

Author details

Hideyuki Komori[1], Ritsuko Iwanaga[2], Andrew P. Bradford[3], Keigo Araki[4] and Kiyoshi Ohtani[4*]

1 Life Sciences Institute, University of Michigan, Ann Arbor, MI, USA

2 Department of Pediatrics, University of Colorado School of Dental Medicine, Aurora, CO, USA

3 Department of Obstetrics and Gynecology, University of Colorado School of Medicine, Aurora, CO, USA

4 Department of Biomedical Chemistry, Kwansei Gakuin University, Sanda, Hyogo, Japan

*Address all correspondence to: btm88939@kwansei.ac.jp

References

[1] Muller H, Helin K. The E2F transcription factors: Key regulators of cell proliferation. Biochimica et Biophysica Acta. 2000;**1470**:1-12

[2] Nevins JR et al. Role of the Rb/E2F pathway in cell growth control. Journal of Cellular Physiology. 1997;**173**:233-236

[3] Chen HZ, Tsai SY, Leone G. Emerging roles of E2Fs in cancer: An exit from cell cycle control. Nature Reviews. Cancer. 2009;**9**:785-797

[4] Dimova DK, Dyson NJ. The E2F transcriptional network: Old acquaintances with new faces. Oncogene. 2005;**24**:2810-2826

[5] Sherr CJ, McCormick F. The RB and p53 pathways in cancer. Cancer Cell. 2002;**2**:103-112

[6] Weng L et al. Critical role of active repression by E2F and Rb proteins in endoreplication during drosophila development. The EMBO Journal. 2003;**22**:3865-3875

[7] Shan B, Lee WH. Deregulated expression of E2F-1 induces S-phase entry and leads to apoptosis. Molecular and Cellular Biology. 1994;**14**:8166-8173

[8] Jiang H et al. The RB-E2F1 pathway regulates autophagy. Cancer Research. 2010;**70**:7882-7893

[9] Muller H et al. E2Fs regulate the expression of genes involved in differentiation, development, proliferation, and apoptosis. Genes & Development. 2001;**15**:267-285

[10] Komori H et al. Distinct E2F-mediated transcriptional program regulates $p14^{ARF}$ gene expression. The EMBO Journal. 2005;**24**:3724-3736

[11] Ozono E et al. E2F-like elements in $p27^{Kip1}$ promoter specifically sense deregulated E2F activity. Genes to Cells. 2009;**14**:89-99

[12] Ozono E et al. Tumor suppressor *TAp73* gene specifically responds to deregulated E2F activity in human normal fibroblasts. Genes to Cells. 2012;**17**:660-672

[13] Komori H et al. Differential requirement for dimerization partner DP between E2F-dependent activation of tumor suppressor and growth-related genes. Scientific Reports. 2018;**8**:8438

[14] Ikeda MA, Jakoi L, Nevins JR. A unique role for the Rb protein in controlling E2F accumulation during cell growth and differentiation. Proceedings of the National Academy of Sciences of the United States of America. 1996;**93**:3215-3220

[15] Gaubatz S et al. E2F4 and E2F5 play an essential role in pocket protein-mediated G1 control. Molecular Cell. 2000;**6**:729-735

[16] Takahashi Y, Rayman JB, Dynlacht BD. Analysis of promoter binding by the E2F and pRB families in vivo: Distinct E2F proteins mediate activation and repression. Genes & Development. 2000;**14**:804-816

[17] Trimarchi JM et al. E2F-6, a member of the E2F family that can behave as a transcriptional repressor. Proceedings of the National Academy of Sciences of the United States of America. 1998;**95**(6):2850-2855

[18] Cartwright P et al. E2F-6: A novel member of the E2F family is an inhibitor of E2F-dependent transcription. Oncogene. 1998;**17**:611-623

[19] Morkel M et al. An E2F-like repressor of transcription. Nature. 1997;**390**:567-568

[20] Okuda M et al. The interaction mode of the acidic region of the cell cycle transcription factor DP1 with TFIIH. Journal of Molecular Biology. 2016;**428**:4993-5006

[21] Qiao H et al. Human TFDP3, a novel DP protein, inhibits DNA binding and transactivation by E2F. The Journal of Biological Chemistry. 2007;**282**:454-466

[22] Milton A et al. A functionally distinct member of the DP family of E2F subunits. Oncogene. 2006;**25**:3212-3218

[23] Kovesdi I, Reichel R, Nevins JR. Role of an adenovirus E2 promoter binding factor in E1A-mediated coordinate gene control. Proceedings of the National Academy of Sciences of the United States of America. 1987;**84**:2180-2184

[24] de Bruin A et al. Identification and characterization of E2F7, a novel mammalian E2F family member capable of blocking cellular proliferation. The Journal of Biological Chemistry. 2003;**278**:42041-42049

[25] Di Stefano L, Jensen MR, Helin K. E2F7, a novel E2F featuring DP-independent repression of a subset of E2F-regulated genes. The EMBO Journal. 2003;**22**:6289-6298

[26] Logan N et al. E2F-7: A distinctive E2F family member with an unusual organization of DNA-binding domains. Oncogene. 2004;**23**:5138-5150

[27] Christensen J et al. Characterization of E2F8, a novel E2F-like cell-cycle regulated repressor of E2F-activated transcription. Nucleic Acids Research. 2005;**33**:5458-5470

[28] Logan N et al. E2F-8: An E2F family member with a similar organization of DNA-binding domains to E2F-7. Oncogene. 2005;**24**:5000-5004

[29] Maiti B et al. Cloning and characterization of mouse E2F8, a novel mammalian E2F family member capable of blocking cellular proliferation. The Journal of Biological Chemistry. 2005;**280**:18211-18220

[30] Kim M, Tang JP, Moon NS. An alternatively spliced form affecting the marked box domain of drosophila E2F1 is required for proper cell cycle regulation. PLoS Genetics. 2018;**14**:e1007204

[31] Royzman I, Whittaker AJ, Orr-Weaver TL. Mutations in drosophila DP and E2F distinguish G1-S progression from an associated transcriptional program. Genes & Development. 1997;**11**:1999-2011

[32] Frolov MV et al. Functional antagonism between E2F family members. Genes & Development. 2001;**15**:2146-21460

[33] Lammens T et al. Atypical E2Fs: New players in the E2F transcription factor family. Trends in Cell Biology. 2009;**19**:111-118

[34] Johnson DG, Ohtani K, Nevins JR. Autoregulatory control of E2F1 expression in response to positive and negative regulators of cell cycle progression. Genes & Development. 1994;**8**:1514-1525

[35] Slansky JE et al. A protein synthesis-dependent increase in E2F1 mRNA correlates with growth regulation of the dihydrofolate reductase promoter. Molecular and Cellular Biology. 1993;**13**:1610-1618

[36] Wu L et al. The E2F1-3 transcription factors are essential for cellular proliferation. Nature. 2001;**414**:457-462

[37] Sharma N et al. Control of the p53-p21CIP1 Axis by E2f1, E2f2, and E2f3 is essential for G1/S progression and cellular transformation. The Journal of Biological Chemistry. 2006;**281**:36124-36131

[38] Timmers C et al. E2f1, E2f2, and E2f3 control E2F target expression and cellular proliferation via a p53-dependent negative feedback loop. Molecular and Cellular Biology. 2007;**27**:65-78

[39] Aslanian A et al. Repression of the Arf tumor suppressor by E2F3 is required for normal cell cycle kinetics. Genes & Development. 2004;**18**:1413-1422

[40] Sage J et al. Acute mutation of retinoblastoma gene function is sufficient for cell cycle re-entry. Nature. 2003;**424**:223-228

[41] Ohtani K, DeGregori J, Nevins JR. Regulation of the cyclin E gene by transcription factor E2F1. Proceedings of the National Academy of Sciences of the United States of America. 1995;**92**:12146-12150

[42] Magnaghi-Jaulin L et al. Retinoblastoma protein represses transcription by recruiting a histone deacetylase. Nature. 1998;**391**:601-605

[43] Luo RX, Postigo AA, Dean DC. Rb interacts with histone deacetylase to repress transcription. Cell. 1998;**92**:463-473

[44] Brehm A et al. Retinoblastoma protein recruits histone deacetylase to repress transcription. Nature. 1998;**391**:597-601

[45] Trouche D et al. RB and hbrm cooperate to repress the activation functions of E2F1. Proceedings of the National Academy of Sciences of the United States of America. 1997;**94**:11268-11273

[46] Nielsen SJ et al. Rb targets histone H3 methylation and HP1 to promoters. Nature. 2001;**412**:561-565

[47] Strobeck MW et al. BRG-1 is required for RB-mediated cell cycle arrest. Proceedings of the National Academy of Sciences of the United States of America. 2000;**97**:7748-7753

[48] Girling R et al. A new component of the transcription factor DRTF1/E2F. Nature. 1993;**365**:468

[49] Helin K et al. Heterodimerization of the transcription factors E2F-1 and DP-1 leads to cooperative transactivation. Genes & Development. 1993;**7**:1850-1861

[50] Zheng N et al. Structural basis of DNA recognition by the heterodimeric cell cycle transcription factor E2F-DP. Genes & Development. 1999;**13**:666-674

[51] Morrison SJ, Kimble J. Asymmetric and symmetric stem-cell divisions in development and cancer. Nature. 2006;**441**:1068-1074

[52] Maehara K et al. Reduction of total E2F/DP activity induces senescence-like cell cycle arrest in cancer cells lacking functional pRB and p53. The Journal of Cell Biology. 2005;**168**:553-560

[53] Tsai SY et al. Mouse development with a single E2F activator. Nature. 2008;**454**:1137-1141

[54] Chen D et al. Division and apoptosis of E2f-deficient retinal progenitors. Nature. 2009;**462**:925-929

[55] Liu H et al. Redeployment of Myc and E2f1-3 drives Rb-deficient cell cycles. Nature Cell Biology. 2015;**17**:1036-1048

[56] Kohn MJ et al. *Dp1* is largely dispensable for embryonic development. Molecular and Cellular Biology. 2004;**24**:7197-7205

[57] Kohn MJ et al. *Dp1* is required for extra-embryonic development. Development. 2003;**130**:1295-1305

[58] Duronio RJ et al. The transcription factor E2F is required for S phase during *Drosophila* embryogenesis. Genes & Development. 1995;**9**:1445-1455

[59] Guarner A et al. E2F/DP prevents cell-cycle progression in endocycling fat body cells by suppressing dATM expression. Developmental Cell. 2017;**43**:689-703 e5

[60] Zappia MP, Frolov MV. E2F function in muscle growth is necessary and sufficient for viability in drosophila. Nature Communications. 2016;**7**:10509

[61] Liu B et al. Interaction of E2F7 transcription factor with E2F1 and C-terminal-binding protein (CtBP) provides a mechanism for E2F7-dependent transcription repression. The Journal of Biological Chemistry. 2013;**288**:24581-24589

[62] Morgunova E et al. Structural insights into the DNA-binding specificity of E2F family transcription factors. Nature Communications. 2015;**6**:10050

[63] Chen HZ et al. Canonical and atypical E2Fs regulate the mammalian endocycle. Nature Cell Biology. 2012;**14**:1192-1202

[64] Orr-Weaver TL. When bigger is better: The role of polyploidy in organogenesis. Trends in Genetics. 2015;**31**:307-315

[65] Zielke N et al. Control of *Drosophila* endocycles by E2F and CRL4(CDT2). Nature. 2011;**480**:123-127

[66] Weiss A et al. Continuous Cyclin E expression inhibits progression through endoreduplication cycles in drosophila. Current Biology. 1998;**8**:239-242

[67] Follette PJ, Duronio RJ, O'Farrell PH. Fluctuations in cyclin E levels are required for multiple rounds of endocycle S phase in *Drosophila*. Current Biology. 1998;**8**:235-238

[68] Bates S et al. p14ARF links the tumour suppressors RB and p53. Nature. 1998;**395**:124-125

[69] Lissy NA et al. A common E2F-1 and p73 pathway mediates cell death induced by TCR activation. Nature. 2000;**407**:642-645

[70] Irwin M et al. Role for the p53 homologue p73 in E2F-1-induced apoptosis. Nature. 2000;**407**:645-648

[71] de Stanchina E et al. E1A signaling to p53 involves the p19^{ARF} tumor suppressor. Genes & Development. 1998;**12**:2434-2442

[72] Lowe SW, Ruley HE. Stabilization of the p53 tumor suppressor is induced by adenovirus 5 E1A and accompanies apoptosis. Genes & Development. 1993;**7**:535-545

[73] Samuelson AV et al. p400 is required for E1A to promote apoptosis. The Journal of Biological Chemistry. 2005;**280**:21915-21923

[74] Hallstrom TC, Nevins JR. Specificity in the activation and control of transcription factor E2F-dependent apoptosis. Proceedings of the National Academy of Sciences of the United States of America. 2003;**100**:10848-10853

[75] Hallstrom TC, Mori S, Nevins JR. An E2F1-dependent gene expression program that determines the balance between proliferation and cell death. Cancer Cell. 2008;**13**:11-22

[76] Kurayoshi K et al. The phosphatidyl inositol 3 kinase pathway does not suppress activation of the *ARF* and *BIM* genes by deregulated E2F1 activity. Biochemical and Biophysical Research Communications. 2017;**482**:784-790

[77] Hallstrom TC, Nevins JR. Jab1 is a specificity factor for E2F1-induced apoptosis. Genes & Development. 2006;**20**:613-623

[78] Lu H et al. Jab1/CSN5 mediates E2F dependent expression of mitotic and apoptotic but not DNA replication targets. Cell Cycle. 2011;**10**:3317-3326

[79] Jacks T et al. Effects of an *Rb* mutation in the mouse. Nature. 1992;**359**:295-300

[80] Tsai KY et al. Mutation of *E2f-1* suppresses apoptosis and inappropriate S phase entry and extends survival of *Rb*-deficient mouse embryos. Molecular Cell. 1998;**2**:293-304

[81] Tsai KY et al. *ARF* mutation accelerates pituitary tumor development in $Rb^{+/-}$ mice. Proceedings of the National Academy of Sciences of the United States of America. 2002;**99**:16865-16870

[82] Yamasaki L et al. Loss of E2F-1 reduces tumorigenesis and extends the lifespan of $Rb1^{+/-}$ mice. Nature Genetics. 1998;**18**:360-364

[83] Moon NS, Di Stefano L, Dyson N. A gradient of epidermal growth factor receptor signaling determines the sensitivity of rbf1 mutant cells to E2F-dependent apoptosis. Molecular and Cellular Biology. 2006;**26**:7601-7615

[84] Myster DL, Bonnette PC, Duronio RJ. A role for the DP subunit of the E2F transcription factor in axis determination during *Drosophila* oogenesis. Development. 2000;**127**:3249-3261

[85] Du W, Xie JE, Dyson N. Ectopic expression of dE2F and dDP induces cell proliferation and death in the drosophila eye. The EMBO Journal. 1996;**15**:3684-3692

[86] Moon NS et al. E2F and p53 induce apoptosis independently during *Drosophila* development but intersect in the context of DNA damage. PLoS Genetics. 2008;**4**:e1000153

[87] Kent LN et al. *E2f8* mediates tumor suppression in postnatal liver development. The Journal of Clinical Investigation. 2016;**126**:2955-2969

[88] Thurlings I et al. Synergistic functions of E2F7 and E2F8 are critical to suppress stress-induced skin cancer. Oncogene. 2017;**36**:829-839

[89] Takahashi K, Yamanaka S. Induction of pluripotent stem cells from mouse embryonic and adult fibroblast cultures by defined factors. Cell. 2006;**126**:663-676

[90] Marion RM et al. A p53-mediated DNA damage response limits reprogramming to ensure iPS cell genomic integrity. Nature. 2009;**460**:1149-1153

[91] Hong H et al. Suppression of induced pluripotent stem cell generation by the p53-p21 pathway. Nature. 2009;**460**:1132-1135

[92] Pajcini KV et al. Transient inactivation of *Rb* and *ARF* yields regenerative cells from postmitotic mammalian muscle. Cell Stem Cell. 2010;**7**:198-213